INTERMITTENT FASTING FOR WOMEN OVER 50

Lose Weight and Prevent Diabetes by Resetting Your Metabolism, Detox Your Body, and Increasing Your Energy and Longevity With Delicious Recipes and 21 Day Meal Plan. Includes a Digital Gift

Arline Hobbs

TABLE OF CONTENTS

A GIFT FOR YOU

Hello thank you for purchasing my book! I thought I'd give a gift to all the readers of my books:

Click on the link and immediately download the

"Keto Diet + 60 recipes + 21 day meal plan"

When you finish reading the book, I would appreciate you leaving an honest review and letting other people know about my books.

It's quick and easy to leave a review, just click on the LINK, and you will automatically go to the reviews section

Thank you for your time and good "Intermittent Fasting"

CHAPTER 1:

What Is Intermittent Fasting?

In recent days, intermittent fasting has become very popular in the fitness community and is also a health trend. Followers of this trend argue that intermittent fasting causes weight loss, improved metabolic health, and, in some cases, intermittent fasting also extends the life span. There are many eating methods, but finding out the correct method that can be effective and work the best for you depends on the individual and can be a bit of a task. There are a lot of methods in this eating pattern, but it is better that you consult a health professional before starting intermittent fasting or deciding how often you should fast.

One thing that has to be kept in mind if you are planning to start your intermittent diet is to eat healthy foods during your eating window. If you eat an excessive number of calories and lots of processed food, this eating method will not work for you, and you will not get any positive results. Just make sure that you eat healthy, balanced food when you are not fasting.

People all over the world are following this method to become healthier by losing weight and improving their lifestyle. In fact, experts believe that following this fasting technique might benefit your brain and your body. During the fasting period, you either have to eat very little or maybe nothing at all to get the best results. By following intermittent fasting and reducing your calorie intake when you are eating, you might be able to lose weight easily.

But also, remember that not everyone can follow intermittent fasting. If you have an eating disorder or you are already very weak and underweight or even pregnant, you should consult your doctor before following this eating method. Make sure that you are well informed or else, it can be downright harmful to you.

Here are some facts that you need to know before you start this eating method –

Intermittent Fasting Definition

Intermittent fasting is the eating pattern where you eat for a specified amount of time in a day and fast for the rest of the day and thus follow a cycle of eating and fasting. This method does not specifically tell you what to eat and what not to eat; rather, it is a pattern of eating where the time when you are eating your food matters. Thus, terming intermitted fasting as a diet would be wrong. Intermittent fasting can be described as a pattern of eating. Mostly in an intermittent fasting method, you will have to follow 16-hours fasting daily or 24 hours twice every week.

Throughout the time that humans have evolved, fasting has been a practice that everyone has followed. Even in ancient times, hunter-gatherers did not have food available all the time. They did not have supermarkets or refrigerators where they could get food available all the time. In fact, there were times when they could not find anything to eat. Thus, humans have evolved in a way that they can function without food for a good amount of time. People think that it is natural to eat 3 to 4 meals a day, but that is not true.

Fasting is also a widespread practice in all religions for spiritual reasons. Religions like Christianity, Hinduism, Islam, Judaism, and Buddhism follow fasting as a ritual. There are a lot of different ways to do intermittent fasting. In all these methods, days or weeks are scheduled according to eating and fasting time. Intermittent fasting also helps in boosting your metabolism. Thus, it helps in staying fit as you eat fewer calories per day.

Intermittent fasting is an eating pattern where your meals are scheduled in a way so that you get the most out of every meal that you eat. As mentioned earlier, intermittent fasting does not tell you what to eat; intermittent fasting tells you when to eat and when to fast. Most of the people, who follow this eating pattern, follow this to reduce weight. By following intermittent fasting, you can get lean and slimmer in just a few days without going on a strict diet and cutting out on a huge amount of calories.

Types of Intermittent Fasting

There are various types of intermittent fasting, but the most effective ones among those are –

The 5:2 Schedule	This is a pattern of intermittent fasting where you can eat healthy and nutritious food five days a week and fast for the other two days a week. On the two days of the week when you are fasting, you have to fast for the majority portion of the day and consume only between 500 to 600 calories per day. This type of intermittent fasting is also known as the Fast Diet and is known to have been popularized by a British journalist named Michael Mosley. In this particular intermittent fasting method, women are recommended to eat around 500 calories, and men are required to eat around 600 calories. For example, you can eat a normal healthy meal five days a week, but the other two days, you have to eat small portions of the meal and two meals of 250 calories for women each day and 300 calories for men each day.
The 16/8 Method	In this fasting pattern, you are recommended to fast every day for approximately 16 hours and eat healthy food for only 8 hours a day. Restricting your eating window for 8 hours a day is an important part of this method. It is totally up to you as to how many meals you want to include in your 8 hours of

	eating window but make sure to eat healthy food which a low in fat and sugar. This method of fasting is the easiest among all as you can have your dinner early, skip your breakfast, and fast till you have your lunch the next morning. For example, you can have your dinner by 8 p.m and easily have your lunch in the afternoon. If you are someone who has a problem with skipping your breakfast and feels hungry in the morning, then this method might be a little hard to get used to, but once you get used to this method, it might work wonders for you. If you are a beginner, drink coffee and water and other such zero-calorie beverages during your fasting hours, which might help you reduce your hunger and cravings. But, as mentioned earlier, do not forget to eat healthy during the 8 hours of the day. This fasting method will not work for you if you do not follow a healthy diet and keep eating processed and junk food and a huge amount of calories during your eating window.
Eat Stop Eat	This method includes fasting once or twice a week for 24 hours. Fitness expert Brad Pilon had popularized this method of intermittent fasting, and this has been popular for quite some years now. If you want to follow this pattern, then you could fast from breakfast one day to breakfast the next day, and that you help you fast for a total period of 24 hours. For example, you could finish your dinner by 7 p.m one day and have your dinner the next day at

	7 p.m. Or, if you want, you could also fast from one breakfast to breakfast the next day. The main aim is to fast for 24 hours, you can do it according to you, and it will give you the same end results.
	If you follow this particular eating pattern to reduce weight, you should remember to stick to your regular diet during the timer that you are eating your meals. You have to limit your calorie intake even when you are not fasting at all. The only downside of this method could be fasting for 24 hours. 24-hour fasting can be very difficult for many people; thus, if you are a beginner, you can start by fasting for 14 hours and then increase the fasting period slowly.
Alternate Day Fasting	In this pattern of fasting, you have to fast almost every other day of the week. There are a lot of methods by which you can follow this fasting pattern. Some people eat about 500 calories during the fasting days. But, some studies also show that most people have not been able to lose weight by following this alternate-day fasting method and also could not maintain their weight than a typical calorie-restrictive diet.
	If you are a beginner, it is better that you stay away from this diet, as fasting every other day can be a bit extreme for you. This diet pattern can make you go to bed very hungry most several days every week. Thus, this diet is not very pleasant and sustainable for the long term.

The Warrior Diet	This particular intermittent fasting pattern was popularized by Ori Hofmekler, who is a great fitness expert. In this diet pattern, you are supposed to eat a small number of raw fruits and vegetables during the day and a big meal at night. It is a pattern where you fast all day and feast at night. This diet gives you a 4-hour eating window. The warrior diet was the first most accepted and popular form of intermittent fasting pattern. The food choice in this diet is mostly similar to the paleo diet, which includes mostly whole, unprocessed food.
Spontaneous Meal Skipping	This eating pattern does not have any structure, and you do not need to follow any particular fasting plan to reap benefits. You could simply skip meals whenever you do not feel hungry or too busy to cook and eat. People who follow this pattern eat every few hours, or they may lose muscles. For this pattern, you could skip your breakfast one day if you do not feel hungry and eat healthy lunch and dinner later. Or if you are traveling and do not find anything to eat, then you could also do a short fast. When you skip two meals in a day spontaneously, you are following the spontaneous intermittent fasting pattern. The only thing that you need to keep in mind is to eat healthy throughout the other time of the day when you are

	eating, or else you could never lose weight by doing any kind of intermittent fasting.

Debunking Intermittent Fasting Myths

Intermittent fasting has become very common these days. This dietary pattern that cycles around fasting and eating is often promoted as a miracle diet. But, there are a lot of myths about intermittent fasting –

- One of the most ongoing myths is that skipping breakfast makes you fat. People commonly believe that the most important meal in a day is breakfast and excessive hunger, cravings, and weight gain are all results of skipping breakfast. But the truth is, skipping breakfast does not make you gain weight, though it may vary from person to person. Thus, breakfast can benefit some people, but it is not essential for your health. In fact, studies have shown that there was no difference in the weight loss between those who eat breakfast and those who skip it.

- Eating smaller meals more often does not increase your metabolism and does not help your body burn more calories. Your body indeed expends some calories by digesting meals, known as the thermic effect of food. But on average, the thermic effect of food only uses around 10% of your total calorie intake. Studies also show that increasing or decreasing meal frequency does not affect total calories burned.

- Another myth is that eating frequently helps by reducing your hunger and keeping your cravings at a limit. But no evidence shows that if you keep on eating more often, it reduces your hunger overall. Some studies also show that you can get more hungry if you keep on eating at frequent intervals.

- The most common myth among people is that your brain needs a regular supply of dietary glucose. But the fact is your body can produce its glucose and fuel your brain, and thus you do not need constant dietary glucose.

- People also believe that intermittent fasting puts your body into a starvation mood, but that is not true. Short-term fasting up to 48 hours increases your metabolism and helps you stay fit and healthy.

- There is also no evidence to show that intermittent fasting makes you lose your muscles. In fact, intermittent fasting helps you maintain muscle mass while dieting.

Who Should Not Be Following Intermittent Fasting?

As mentioned earlier, people have different needs, and every body type is different. So consult your doctor or nutritionist before following this eating pattern.

Here are few reasons why people suffering from various health conditions should not try intermittent fasting –

- You should avoid intermittent fasting if you have higher caloric needs. If you are already underweight and struggling with weight gain, intermittent fasting is not a good option. Your body needs sufficient calories, and thus, you should avoid such eating patterns daily.

- You should also avoid intermittent fasting if you do not want to feel dehydrated, feel tired, feel hungry, overeat or become irritable. Intermittent fasting is also not for faint-hearted people, and thus if you are someone who has cardiovascular issues, you should avoid this eating pattern.

- You should also avoid intermittent fasting if you are suffering from eating disorders like bulimia nervosa; you should not follow intermittent fasting.

9

Frequently Asked Questions

Here are a few most frequently asked questions about intermittent fasting –

Will I break my fast if I drink liquids?

You can drink water, coffee, and any other type of zero-calorie beverage. Just make sure that you are not adding any extra sugar to your coffee; rather, a small amount of cream might be alright. Experts also recommend having coffee during fasting as it can help you control your cravings.

Should I skip my breakfast?

As mentioned earlier, skipping your breakfast is not unhealthy. The only problem is that the most stereotypical breakfast-skippers fall sick because they have an unhealthy lifestyle. It will not matter if you skip your breakfast as long as you make sure that you are eating healthy food whenever you are eating. You can follow any eating pattern you want; just make sure that you are eating healthy.

Can I take my supplements when I am fasting?

Yes, it is completely fine and safe for you to take supplements while you are fasting. Just make sure to consult with your doctor and check if you can take your vitamin supplements as some vitamins that are fat-soluble might give you better results when it is taken before or after a meal.

Can I do my daily exercise when I am fasting?

Yes, it is completely normal for you to exercise during fasting. Some experts recommend that if you take branched-chain amino acids (BCAAs) during fasting before work out, you might get better results and also be able to work out properly without feeling weak.

Does fasting cause muscle loss?

People often ask this question, and almost every other person is worried about losing their muscles. The truth is every weight loss practice can lead to muscle loss, and so it is important for you to keep lifting weights and also keep consuming a high amount of protein during the part of the day when you are eating. In fact, one of the research also shows that intermittent fasting causes lesser muscle loss than other weight loss methods.

If I follow intermittent fasting, will my metabolism slow down?

No. This is a completely wrong concept. In fact, studies show that short-term regular fasting can actually help you stay fit and boost your metabolism. On the other hand, it is also true that if you fast for a long time, longer than three or more days, then it can be bad for your health. Fasting for a long time can have an adverse effect on your life and health and can suppress your metabolism.

Is it okay for kids to fast?

No. Do not let your child fast. Children below the age of 18 years should not be allowed to fast as it is their growing years; they need all the nutrients to grow and for the proper development of their body. Thus, letting children fast is a bad idea.

What to Eat and What to Avoid During Intermittent Fasting?

Intermittent fasting can be an effective way of losing weight and keep you fit and healthy. But intermittent fasting can only prove to be effective when you know what to eat and what to avoid while following this eating pattern. An intermittent diet does not mandate any specific menus. But here is a list of food items that you should include in your intermittent fasting diet –

- Include lean protein in your diet. Eating lean protein is better than having other things as it keeps you full for a longer time and also helps you to build or maintain your muscles. You could include chicken breast, plain Greek yogurt, beans, peas, lentils, all kinds of fish, shellfish, tofu, and tempeh in your intermittent fasting diet. These are a good source of healthy and lean protein.

- Including fruits of any kind in the diet regime is important. Fruits are packed with plenty of nutrients like vitamins, minerals, phytonutrients, and fiber, keeping you healthy and fit. Vitamins and minerals help lower your cholesterol levels, control your blood pressure, and maintain your bowel health. Include fruits like apricot, apple, blueberries, cherries, peaches, pears, plums, oranges, melons, etc., to your diet will be great as fruits are low in calories and great food options to consume during intermittent fasting.

- Also, include vegetables in your intermittent fasting diet. Vegetables can be an important part of your diet. Research shows that including green leafy vegetables in your diet might reduce heart disease, diabetes, and cancer risk. Vegetables like carrots, broccoli, tomatoes, cauliflower, green beans, kale, spinach, chard, cabbage, collard greens, and arugula can help you stay fit and is also an excellent choice as they supply a lot of nutrients and fiber.

There are also a few things that you should avoid if your aim is to reduce weight and stay fit by following intermittent fasting. Your eating window should be filled with all good food and not junk food. You should stop eating food that contains a huge amount of calories, contain a high amount of added sugar, and avoid having food that contains a high level of saturated fats and salt. That can be very unhealthy for your heart health. These foods do not contain many nutrients and are very harmful to your body.

Here is a list of few things that you should stop eating if you are following intermittent fasting –

- Cookies
- Snacks chips
- Pretzels
- Crackers
- Candy
- Cakes

- Fruit drinks that have added sugar

- Coffees and teas that have added sugar

- Also, cereals that contain a lot of sugar and very little fiber and granola

These unhealthy foods will not make you feel full for a long time; rather, after eating these junk foods, you might feel hungrier very often. Also, experts say that these food items provide little to no nutrients at all. Avoiding high sugar foods is one of the best things that you can do to stay fit and lose weight. Processed sugar is devoid of nutrition and is not what you seek if you follow intermittent fasting. Sugar metabolizes at a very fast rate and makes you feel hungry very fast.

There are a lot of health risks associated with fasting of any kind. But also, intermittent fasting is one of the great ways to lose weight. Also, some studies have proved that people who follow intermittent fasting have better blood pressure and better heart health, and this method even helps keep diabetes in check. As long as you stick to healthy foods, intermittent fasting can have significant health benefits. If you want to lose weight, this is one of the best ways to improve your metabolism and simplify your life as well.

CHAPTER 2:

How to Calculate Your Ideal BMI?

BMI is a complex medical term, and most of us get confused when we hear such terms. You have probably heard your doctor use this term a lot and might have wondered what BMI actually means. The full form of BMI is body mass index. In simple words, your body weight determines your BMI. But should you be worried about your BMI and your family's BMI as well? Is it that serious?

Definition of BMI

As mentioned earlier, the full form of BMI is body mass index. Most medical professionals use BMI to measure your body weight, and after calculating the BMI, people are categorized as being obese, normal weight, or being overweight.

CDC or Centers for Disease Control and Prevention have used this approach to find out that out of the total population of America, one-third are obese. An estimation had been produced by CDC for the year 2008 where it states that America approximately had spent $147 billion in healthcare that year. Research by the CDC has also shown that an obese person in America spends a lot more than people with normal weight, which is almost $1429 per year.

Although some critics argue that if your BMI is not normal then can have health risk for a few particular diseases and health issues, but BMI is not always perfect. The CDC argues that BMI should not be used as a measurement to define any body type as fat or overweight or thin or too skinny. Rather, the CDC argues that your physician should use low or high BMI to understand if you need health check-ups, for example, high cholesterol level or high blood pressure.

In most cases, if your BMI is high, then it might affect your insurance rate.

Importance of Healthy BMI

A report from the CDC shows that most American adults are obese. A report from 2018 also shows that more than 40 percent, meaning around 90.3 million Americans are obese. Maintaining a healthy BMI can be more important for you if you are an adult, as BMI determines your health to a certain extent. If your BMI is high, then your risk of heart diseases and type 2 diabetes also increases, and thus, you can fall sick really soon in the future.

Thus, if you want to stay fit and stay away from all health risks, then it is better that you get your BMI calculated and then take actions accordingly to stay fit.

How to Calculate Your BMI Properly?

The correct way to calculate your BMI is a very simple process if you know how to do it. All you need to do is take your weight in kgs and divide it by squaring your height (in meters). Make sure to not make any mistakes in calculation, or you will end up having the wrong BMI for yourself. That will be a problem for your health expert to advise you properly.

Let me set an example so that understanding the calculation becomes easy for you. If you are a woman who weighs 63.5 kgs and 1.60 meters in height, then to calculate your BMI, all you have to do is –

- Height in meters squared is 1.60 x 1.60 = 2.56
- Weight divided by squared height = 63.5 / 2.56 = 24.80

Yes, it is that simple. Calculating your actual BMI is that simple. But if maths is not your forte, you could give the basic information like your actual height and weight to someone who is good in maths and tell them to calculate it for you.

A Healthy BMI: A List of Ranges

If your height and weight is near to what I have mentioned in the example just above this, then here is a list of what your BMI number means –

- If your BMI is below 18.5, then you are underweight, and that is not normal

- If your BMI is between 18.5 to 24.9, that means you are normal

- If your BMI ranges between 25 to 29.9, then you are overweight

- If your BMI is 30 or more than that, then you are obese

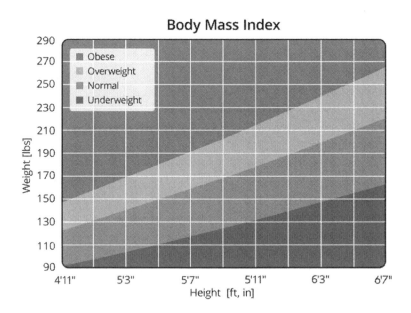

In most cases, the BMI cutoffs are the same, and it does not depend on your gender and age, but in general, women usually have more percentage of body fat than men of the same height and weight. And as we get older, our body weight consists more of body fat than of muscles.

Some people also refer to some charts, which makes it easier for them to calculate their BMI and helps them categorize themselves into healthy, overweight, or obese depending your height and weight. If you have a correct BMI chart with you, you also do not need to calculate your BMI; you could just check your height and weight and understand which category you fall in.

How BMI Affects Your Risks and Longevity

Various studies have shown that higher BMI can be associated with a lot of health issues like –

- Heart disease
- Type 2 diabetes
- Gallbladders diseases
- Cancer
- Depression
- Fatty liver diseases (nonalcoholic)
- Sleep apnea
- Arthritis

The basic cause of your body function malfunctioning is mostly because of higher than normal body weight, which means that your body has a lot of fat which is not good for your body. Stress on organs and bones, rise in blood glucose levels, overproduction of hormones, and formation of plaque in arteries are all caused due to the overproduction of fat cells. That makes your body overwhelmed, and thus, your body does its best to balance itself out.

If you do not consume the proper amount of fruits and vegetables, then your BMI might increase as these foods are less in density than other foods. Having high sugar and fat food will increase your BMI as these have a higher density than vegetables and fruits.

There is also interesting research regarding higher BMI and its effect on chronic diseases. According to some research, if you are hospitalized for some chronic health conditions like heart diseases or cancer, a high BMI might help you survive and protect yourself. Your weight and muscle loss can be compensated by the extra muscle and fat you have accumulated for the loss that you have had due to a serious and life-threatening illness and can also help you in speedy recovery.

How Can You Lower Your BMI?

As your height is fixed, you have to reduce your weight to maintain your BMI. You could make smart food choices like eating a lot of high-fiber and low-calorie food like fruits and vegetables in the correct amount can help you in reducing your weight can maintaining your BMI. Even adding whole grains to your diet is also a proven way to boost your weight loss.

You could also exercise regularly along with consuming nutritious food. Research has shown that a regular workout of 150 minutes can help you in maintaining your BMI. You could include physical activities like swimming, running, and jogging and slowly increase the intensity of your exercise to get better results.

You could also get adequate sleep and manage stress. Lack of sleep can increase the risk of cardiovascular diseases, diabetes, depression, and obesity. Proper sleep also helps in reducing stress to an extent. Chronic stress can also be bad for your health, and some people tend to eat a lot during stress. Thus, find a way to get rid of your chronic stress, and that might help you stay fit and, in turn, help you maintain your BMI.

Intermittent fasting may also boost your weight loss and help you in maintaining your healthy BMI. In intermittent fasting, your meals and snacks get restricted to a strict time window, and that will naturally decrease your calorie intake thus, helping you in weight loss. Intermittent fasting also increases the level of norepinephrine, which helps in boosting your metabolism. This eating pattern also helps maintain your insulin level, which helps keep your blood sugar level under control and can bump up the fat-burning process. Research also shows that intermittent fasting reduces your body weight by 8% and decreases your body fat by 16% in a short period of 2 to 3 weeks.

Flaws in BMI

Research has shown that BMI is not flawless, and it does not take many important factors into account while calculating someone's BMI. Essential factors like activity level, muscle mass, and nutrition also play a huge role in determining if a person is healthy or not. Other approaches that are more appropriate than BMI are –

- Body fat percentage

- Waist to hip ratio

- Waist circumference

- Weight to height ratio

The ideal rate of BMI differs from one race to another; a BMI that is considered healthy for Europeans is considered unhealthy for Asians. Athletes, Asians, and people above the age of 65 may not have the ideal BMI but are still considered healthy by doctors. Also, using the same rate of BMI for men and women is considered wrong by some health experts. Although BMI is used a lot in determining someone's health and categorizing them as fit and unfit, the limitations of BMI make it less useful, and that is why having alternative weight measuring approaches are necessary.

CHAPTER 3:

Benefits of Intermittent Fasting

Intermittent fasting- also referred to as IF- is one of the most effective and sustainable methods for losing weight. There are various ways of intermittent fasting that you can incorporate into your everyday life, as discussed in the first chapter, such as the *daily method*, *alternate method*, the *5:2 method*, or the *24-hour method*. All of these methods work very well for people spanning across different age and gender groups. This chapter will discuss the specific benefits intermittent fasting has for women who fall in the age group over 50.

Unlike popular beliefs, intermittent fasting is a suitable weight-loss method for people in the older age group as well. In fact, there are a bunch of specific health benefits for the people who belong to this age group can achieve from properly practicing intermittent fasting. Dr. Becky, a renowned fitness consultant and physiologist for the over-50 group, states that it is quite difficult to find any disadvantages for intermittent fasting if it is done wisely and not in an extreme manner. She recommends this mode of diet for elderly people as well since it is the one that targets hormone regulation swiftly. That will help burn fat faster than a lot of other weight loss methods, including exercise, which might be a little tougher (but not impossible) to incorporate into your lifestyle if you are in the over-50 age group.

Why Is Intermittent Fasting Suitable for Women Over 50?

Women who are over 50 might face some difficulties in their quest to lose that extra pound of stubborn fat. This does not mean that they should give up, and this is also not a negative indicator in any way. These difficulties can originate from a number of reasons. The main reason is a slower rate of metabolism, which naturally happens due to old age. Our metabolism is a lot faster when we have more lean muscles in our body, but as we get older, the portion of lean muscle mass in our body goes down. This makes it harder for us to get more frequently active with old age and leads to a slower metabolism. The ultimate result is that it becomes harder and harder to get rid of body fat.

Intermittent fasting has become more and more popular for women in this age group due to the fact that it comes with a wide range of benefits besides just weight loss. This method has been demonstrated to be helpful for not just improving your metabolism but also improving your mental health, keep aging at bay, and act as a barrier for certain kinds of cancer. In addition to that, it can also help prevent several nerves, joint, and muscle disorders that women over the age of 50 are easily susceptible to. According to a study published in the Journal of Mid-Life Health, fasting can also be therapeutic for women who belong to this age group.

Is Intermittent Fasting Safe for Older Women?

A lot of older women are wary of adopting intermittent fasting simply out of safety concerns. Although this fear is valid, it also has very little scientific grounding. If done correctly, intermittent fasting can help with excess fat and many other health conditions linked with old age. It also helps older women deal with the changes their bodies go through in terms of their reproductive cycle, which not a lot of other weight loss techniques can vouch for. Plus, due to old age, it becomes harder to do physical exercise for longer times. You might even end up spraining yourself or causing other minor injuries simply owing to the fact that your body is not very well equipped to deal with such workouts anymore. In place of these, intermittent fasting comes in as a much more convenient and safe alternative that can be practiced regardless of age and movement restrictions.

The only potential risks that you might have would have to be due to comorbid medical conditions or in case your body weight is already alarmingly low. However, these are exceptional cases, and even then, intermittent fasting can be your way to go once you have consulted your physician for proper instructions.

Intermittent Fasting and Regulation of Hormones

For women who are aged over 50 years, one of the prime benefits of practicing intermittent fasting is that it helps their rate of metabolism while also helping the regulation of their hormones. There are different metabolic changes which intermittent fasting can help account for among these women. Some of these changes include –

1. **Insulin:** Insulin is a hormone produced in our body by the pancreas. When we are eating, our bodies are tuned to naturally produce this hormone so that it can break down the carbohydrates in the food we eat and turn those into glucose, suited for later use. This glucose is stored in our bodies as fat, which leads to weight gain. What intermittent fasting does is turn this process around effectively. During the period of fasting, the levels of insulin in your body will fall steadily. This will help you improve the rate and the steadiness of how fat is burned by your cells on a regular basis, resulting in a long-term healthy weight loss cycle.

2. **Noradrenaline:** Noradrenaline is a hormone that is produced in our body by our sympathetic nervous system. It controls our blood pressure and can also affect our weight and metabolism. While responding to an empty stomach - which intermittent fasting will help secure for a longer time - your nervous system will send a chemical response to your cells. This will let your cells know that the body needs some

fuel to function, prompting them to release the fat which is already stored in your body. This way, you will also lose fat, along with running your bodily functions smoothly.

3. **HGH:** The pituitary gland is responsible for the production of the human growth hormone, popularly known as HGH, and that can also help you to lose weight through intermittent fasting. The release and functioning of HGH are linked with how insulin functions in our body. HGH is produced as a response in your body when you need glucose. This means that when you are constantly eating, the production of HGH gets stunted, as you are getting all your glucose from external sources. When your insulin levels drop - which happens during prolonged periods of fasting - your HGH levels will increase. This, in turn, will motivate your body to not just grow your muscles but also burn fat. Intermittent fasting has been shown to shoot up HGH production by up to five times its normal rate.

Intermittent Fasting Also Helps With Longevity

Other than simple weight loss benefits, intermittent fasting is also helpful due to the anti-aging effects it can have, specifically for people in the older age group. This way, this fasting technique paves the way for a solution that helps you with both weight loss as well as longevity. Longevity is achieved through a process called autophagy. What happens in autophagy - which is the natural way for our body to clean itself of all the old and damaged cells with new, healthier ones - is that your cells are basically recycled! This does wonders for your longevity because, this way, your body is triggered to produce younger cells a lot faster. This is how intermittent fasting makes way for a healthy and natural way for your body to replenish itself and turn the clocks back on your body while losing steady weight.

Autophagy is an age-old technique, and intermittent fasting is one of the easier ways to get it into your body's natural system. Of course, this system cannot be stretched out for an indefinite amount of time, but that need not be the case since in between periods of fasting, you would also be eating a balanced diet every day (or every other day, depending on the method of fasting which you are following). Intermittent fasting simply increases the rate of autophagy by putting your cells under additional stress. It is not unhealthy if you maintain a steady self-eating cycle, which should be a given if you are practicing intermittent fasting.

Autophagy, where your brain basically clears itself out or 'takes out the trash,' is also great for you because it detoxifies your mind. By clearing out old and damaged cells, intermittent fasting helps fight depression, Alzheimer's disease, and several other neuropsychiatric conditions that are harmful to your brain. Older people are particularly prone to some of these conditions (such as Alzheimer's), which is why this method of weight loss is best suitable for them since it is the easiest way of triggering autophagy in your body.

Intermittent Fasting Has Wonderful Mental Health Benefits

Here are five incredible things intermittent fasting can do to your body which has positive effects on your mental health, which are reasons enough for you to give them a try, even if you are not so hard on the weight loss part –

1. **Helps improve memory:** Intermittent fasting can help you improve your focus and your memory. Limiting the hours during which you are eating can drastically improve concentration and memory, as has been shown by a study published in the Journal of the Academy of Nutrition and Dietetics. In this study, people practiced intermittent fasting for just four weeks and showed signs of considerable improvement in aspects such as working memory and spatial memory, and planning. Other than this, studies have also shown that intermittent fasting improves learning in general.

2. **Lifts up your mood:** If you continue intermittent fasting regularly for a longer period of time (three months or more),

studies have shown that you would start to see several changes in your mood. You would, in general, be happier with an improved overall mood. Plus, you will also notice a fall in the levels of anger, tension, as well as indecisiveness or confusion. Other studies have also shown that intermittent fasting can be associated with great improvements in a person's emotional well-being and help with mental health problems such as depression.

3. **Checks your blood sugar:** Blood sugar rates have been linked with anxiety and depression (apart from health conditions such as diabetes), and it is important for people in the age group over 50 to have a healthy level of blood sugar even for normal day-to-day functioning. Intermittent fasting helps with insulin sensitivity, which in turn helps fight high levels of blood sugar. This has great effects on your brain as it protects you from higher vulnerability towards anxiety and depression, among other things.

4. **Lowers your blood pressure:** Intermittent fasting helps reduce your blood pressure, especially at night when you are catching up on sleep. This is extremely helpful for your heart, but it is also very good for the health of your brain. If your blood pressure is not under control - which is if you are more prone to hypertension - then the blood that flows to your brain will be cut off, and you would run serious health risks. Intermittent fasting helps prevent that. Low blood flow to the brain has been linked to several mental health conditions such as schizophrenia, substance abuse, ADHD, depression, and bipolar disorder. All of these can be kept under check to some extent by regulating your blood pressure.

5. **Reduces the chance of inflammation:** Although this might sound like something which will only help your body, reducing inflammation also has a great positive impact on your brain. Chronic inflammation has been associated with several brain disorders. These include obsessive-compulsive disorder, schizophrenia, and bipolar disorder. According to a study which was published in Nutrition Research,

intermittent fasting can significantly decrease inflammation, which improves the well-being of your brain to a great extent.

Other than all of these targeted benefits, the primary goal of intermittent fasting is to burn excess fat, especially stubborn fat, which is a bigger problem among women over the age of 50. Burning excess body fat can also be very good for your brain and your mental health. Excess fat in your body, which is hard to shed off, can increase the chances of obesity - especially during older ages when the body's normal rate of activity decreases - and that can cause your brain a lot of harm. Weight loss can help keep several mental illnesses such as phobias, addictions, and depressive disorders under check.

Intermittent Fasting Can Be Helpful for Post-Menopausal Women

A lot of women go through menopause around the ages of 50 to 55 years. During this time, women are susceptible to several health conditions- both physical and mental. Due to these complications, it sometimes becomes important for them to expedite their weight loss so that they can keep their metabolism under check. There have been various studies that have shown how a change in diets and fasting techniques can be particularly beneficial when it comes to regulating as well as losing weight for women who are going through or have just gone through menopause.

A study published by the National Library of Medicine proves that different types of intermittent fasting have both short and long-term positive effects for menopausal women. Some of the kinds of intermittent fasting which help the women in this age group, in particular, include eat-stop-eat, the 5/2 and 16/8 methods, and a method known as the warrior diet. These diets not just help keep your weight under check, they also help improve your digestive systems, decrease any chances of inflammation, and reduce overall body fat.

However, you must know that you must avoid intermittent fasting if you have certain health conditions such as heart disease or diabetes, as in these situations, depriving your body of food for longer times might do more harm than good.

This chapter sums up how intermittent fasting can be a powerful tool for people across all demographics and women who belong to the age group above 50. Women of this age often find it harder to lose weight due to the body's slowed down metabolism or other conditions. In such a situation, crash diets, pills, and several other speedy treatments would not work and would worsen both physical and mental health. Intermittent fasting is one of the aptest weight loss methods for women above the age of 50. The chapter has briefly listed out how this strategy can help women with their metabolism, hormones, mental health, and menopause. If you were wondering if intermittent fasting is the right weight loss route for you or were just looking for a method that suits you best, this chapter might just have been the push you needed in the right direction!

CHAPTER 4:

Physical Exercises That Help

Exercise has its own perks. It does not matter what kind of diet you are following or what kind of food habits you have; you have to do some kind of exercise daily. Even if you are following intermittent fasting, it is still important that you maintain your regular workout schedule while fasting. Both intermittent fasting and exercise are practiced by people because they are components of cultivating longevity. Studies have shown that when you combine exercise with intermittent fasting, it raises your hormones and makes you more insulin sensitive, and that is how it helps you to stay fit, young, and lean for a long time.

Some people think that working out without refueling your body can be harmful and can lead to muscle loss. But that is not true. Your body's hormones get a lot of benefits when you work out during fasting. Exercising during fasting has also proved to be a great way to boost your health and body composition.

Things You Should Know

If you are following intermittent fasting, you should keep in mind a few things while working out to make your workout effective and keep you safe during the workout session. Here is a list of things that you should try while continuing your exercise routine during intermittent fasting –

- *When to Workout* – The most common question that people have is when is the right time to work out during intermittent fasting? Should you work out before, during, or after having your meal? One of the most well-known methods of intermittent fasting is the 16:8 method. In this method, you are supposed to eat healthy food during the 8-hour fueling window and fast for the remaining 16 hours. Experts recommend that different exercising methods work for different people. Some do not like to work out on an empty stomach and might not get the time to work out during the fueling window, and such people might like to work out after the eating window. For some people, they can function well on an empty stomach, and that exercising method might be better suited for them and others; working out during the eating window might seem a good option as they might not function well on an empty stomach and also want to capitalize on post-workout nutrition.

- *Choose Your Workout Style Depending on Your Macronutrients* – Gym trainers and fitness experts suggest that you choose your workout style during intermittent fasting depending on the micronutrients you consume to get better results. It is important for you to pay attention to what you are eating before exercising and what you are eating after exercising. For example, if your workout needs strength, then you should consume more carbohydrates, while on the days of cardio, you should consume a low-carb diet to get better results.

- *Choose The Right Meal to Maintain Your Muscle* – Experts suggest that to get the best result, you should combine intermittent fasting and exercise during the eating periods so that your nutrition level is peaked. If you are during heavy weight lifting, then it is important that you eat food that is rich in protein after working out, as that will help you to maintain and build muscles. Experts also suggest that you eat protein after a heavy intensity workout within 30 mins of finishing it. Your diet should also contain high fiber carbs and healthy fats when you are combining intermittent fasting and exercise to get better results. You could eat scrambled eggs with veggies or protein shakes, and protein bars can also work.

- *Hydrate Your Body* – Consuming plenty of water and also electrolytes is very important, especially when you are fasting and working out at the same time. If your body is dehydrated and your electrolytes are not balanced properly, then you could face problems like headaches, dizziness, low blood sugar, low blood pressure, nausea, and cramps. Keep drinking unsweetened coconut water and zero-calorie electrolyte drinks, and if your body becomes very dehydrated, you could also consume electrolyte tablets. But make sure that you are not consuming sports drinks that are high in sugar to stay hydrated, as that will ruin your diet and your workout as well. Along with staying hydrated, also make sure to consume adequate sodium and potassium.

- ***Do Not Start Keto And Intermittent Fasting at The Same Time*** – Your body cannot handle two diets at the same time, give your body some time to get used to one diet and then start another one after a few weeks. Your body needs time to adjust to these new changes, so you could first start keto, where you would consume less amount of carbs before you start intermittent fasting. You might want to stop whatever diet you are following if you feel any mental fog, weakness, dizziness, exhaustion, burnout, injuries, nausea, etc. Also, remember that extra workouts will make you feel hungrier, and thus, fasting will become an impossible task for you, especially if the intensity of your workout is too high.

- ***Listen to Your Body*** – If you are someone who has health issues that causes dizziness, like low blood sugar or low blood pressure, then you should avoid working out during fasting. If you do not feel well, do not make your body go through that pain. Listen to your body and stop right there and do what feels right. You might feel weak during the workout, stop immediately, refuel and hydrate yourself and relax. It is better that you consult your doctor before starting intermittent fasting or working out during fasting, as they can guide you on what is right for you and your body.

- ***Exercising And Intermittent Fasting for Weight Loss*** – The main reason people follow the intermittent fasting method is to lose weight. People also think that if they combine intermittent fasting with a daily workout, it could help them lose weight faster. This can be true in some cases, but this plan may also backfire in some cases. As mentioned earlier, an extra workout can make you feel more hungry and make fasting for you a tough job. To lose weight, you just have to choose a diet that will create a calorie deficit. If you overeat during your eating window, even a workout or intermittent fasting will not help. If your goal is to lose weight, then you need to keep track of what you eat and use portion control. You might also want to choose your workout style and avoid doing high-intensity workouts. Remember that slow and sustainable weight loss is the best kind of weight loss for your body.

Some Common Workouts That You Can And Cannot Do

Here is a list of exercises that you can do while you are following an intermittent diet –

Yoga	Experts recommend people practice yoga on an empty stomach as it provides a clean and light feeling, and your mind can focus entirely on your breath and body's movement. Thus, yoga is one of the best exercises that you can practice during intermittent fasting.
Dance	If you get hungry really fast and following intermittent fasting seems like trouble to you, you could try dancing of any form as an exercise activity as dance is fun and people tend to forget any kind of hunger when they are dancing. You could try Ballet, Zumba, Barre, Hip-hop, etc., to get the best results.
Tennis	People who are avid tennis players often play tennis in the morning when their stomach is empty and the morning breeze is fast. Thus, you could

	also play tennis, and that would be a good exercise for you when you are fasting.
Walking or Jogging	If you are fasting, one of the most useful exercises you could do is walk or fast from anywhere in between 1 to 4 miles. If you are walking on a treadmill, try walking on an incline, as it has proven to be more effective in burning fat and losing weight than jogging.
Cycling	It does not matter whether you are cycling indoors or outdoors; as long as you are enjoying it and cycling for a long time, it can be a very useful exercise for you when you are fasting.
Pilates	Fitness experts recommend people to do pilates when their stomach is empty. Experts prefer a light state of being while practicing pilates as, according to them, that is when you get the best results.

Here is a list of workouts that you should avoid when you are fasting –

- Boxing
- Powerlifting
- CrossFit
- HIIT

Cardio While Fasting

You might be wondering whether you should do cardio on an empty stomach. You might also be wondering if doing cardio on an empty stomach has any fat-burning benefits. People who believe in doing cardio while fasting say that the practice maximizes your fat-burning potential. Fasted cardio can offer you great benefits if you aim to lower your body weight and lower the fat percentage by doing low to moderate-intensity cardio. Even research shows that if you run in the fasted state, then you might burn more fat than when your body does not have circulating nutrients to use for energy. For example, a study shows that when a person ran on a treadmill while fasting, they burned more fat (20% more) compared to those who had eaten before running.

Experts also say that doing fasted cardio regularly helps you to get rid of the stubborn fat easily, which would otherwise take a lot of time to burn. But experts also recommend people who are new at working out not try high-intensity cardio while fasting. People who have been working out for a while know their body limits and know where to stop.

If you think that the benefit of fasted cardio is limited only to body composition changes, you might be wrong. In the initial days when you will start to run on an empty stomach, you might feel sluggish and too tired to do any kind of work, but with time, you will get used to it, and you will love doing it because you will be able to see results and understand how efficient doing cardio while fasting is.

Experts suggest that this exercising technique becomes more effective and seems more beneficial when you start working out for more than 30 minutes. Research published in the journal of Applied Physiology has also shown that people who have been doing cardio while fasting has lost more weight and burned more fat than those who ate properly before working out when both of these group of people trained at the same intensity.

Thus most people skip their meals, especially breakfast, before working out as it gives them a better result and helps them to burn fat easily. In fact, most of the fitness experts recommend people to wait at least 30 mins after having their meal before working out, but 30 minutes of standard time is recommended when the meal is really light like a banana, or a boiled egg, or a slice of toast with nut butter. But the best way is to work out on an empty stomach and wait to eat until after your workout to achieve your desired body weight faster.

Here are some tips for you if you are doing fasted cardio as following these few rules can help you to stay safe –

- It is recommended that you do not exceed your cardio workout time for more than 60 minutes when you are fasting.

- If you are new at fasted cardio, it is better that you choose low to moderate intensity workouts and do not overdo anything that will e too much for your body to take.

- You have to stay hydrated, and that is the key to fasted cardio, keep drinking water or other zero-calorie drinks to stop your body from getting dehydrated.

- Remember that your lifestyle and the amount your nutrition that you are consuming play a huge role in determining whether you will lose weight and stay fit by following fasted cardio or will it not be of any help to your body at all.

As mentioned earlier, the key to staying fit and not falling sick by following fasted cardio is listening to your body and doing what you feel is the best for you. You could also consult your doctor, personal trainer, dietician if you have any questions regarding fasted cardio and to find out if this method will be fine for your body as well.

Exercise Routines to Try

Here is a list of exercise routines that you could try if you want to exercise during intermittent fasting –

- *A routine you can try if you have 30 minutes* – You could go out for a 15 minutes walk and walk for at least one mile in that 15 minutes, or you could also try walking on an incline on a treadmill. For the other 15 minutes, you could do some bodyweight exercises like core workout, pushups, squats, lunges, etc.

- *A routine you can try if you have 45 minutes* – You could walk or jog outside for 20 to 30 minutes and cover a distance of at least 2 miles, or you could also try to walk on an incline on a treadmill and that will give you the same benefits. After walking or jogging for 30 minutes, you could spend the following 15 minutes practicing through yoga vinyasas, or you could also practice bodyweight exercises mentioned above. Choosing the kind of workout you want to do totally depends on you and differs from one individual to another, so do what seems best for your body.

- *A routine you can try if you have 1 hour* – If you can afford a time period of one hour daily for your exercise, then you could check what exercise classes ate available in your locality, or you could go for a bike ride, or could also taker a long walk in the park. You could also ask your friend to join you, and you could walk and ride a bicycle with your friend, or you could also take up swimming classes. You could also turn on a movie and spend an hour while walking on the treadmill on an incline. In this way, you would be able to catch up on your favorite shows and movies while working out.

All you have to do is keep moving and get your workout done. Also, remember to stay hydrated and stop immediately if you feel week or dizzy and feel like you are going to faint. It is completely okay to work out while following intermittent fasting because you cannit lose weight and gain muscle only by following a certain eating method; you need to work out daily for hormone optimization. Studies have shown that following intermittent fasting alone can be very amazing for your body, but when you combine intermittent fasting with exercise, it can work wonders, and you might get a whole new level of benefits.

CHAPTER 5:

Practice Meditation

Our busy lifestyle comes in the way of our dietary habits. We seldom find time to eat wholesome homemade food or sometimes even skip meals due to our work schedule. This is one big reason why despite investing a good amount of money on commercial diets every month, some people do not get the desired results.

Following a diet requires discipline, wisdom, and love for self to be able to meet daily goals. We must become more mindful, slow down, especially while planning and preparing our meals when eating and moving during the day. This will help us be more aware of the kind of food we are consuming and any malpractice that keeps us from losing those extra pounds. A very good way of attaining this consciousness needed by our minds is to practice meditation every day, even if for a few minutes.

How Meditation Helps In Building a Healthier Relationship With Food

Let us learn how meditation can help us in our weight loss journey. Experts believe that our body is the mirror to our thoughts; that is, our body can tell a lot about what is going on in our minds. The weight loss journey can feel burdensome and exhausting if we do not take a psychological approach to the process. Sometimes people who have faced traumas or have had mental health issues in the past are likely to have an unhealthy relationship with food that has resulted in their present body condition. Meditation helps with this. It allows you to be in touch with your inner self, understand your feelings, confront your thoughts, learn how you perceive yourself, and realize how much you love and care about yourself. Therefore, meditation helps us to have a better understanding of the reason for the weight showing up.

Meditation for weight loss involves walking in a peaceful atmosphere, lying, sitting, focusing attention on a word maybe or through breathing techniques, and being open to assess what you learn. Doing as minimum as sitting in a quiet place enables us to relax and reflect on our health and the habits that are acting as a hindrance or beneficial in attaining better health. It helps us concentrate on our thoughts and enter a dialogue with our minds questioning the reason for indulging in the junk food we eat. It enables us to identify the roots of the problems that are making it difficult to follow a weight loss program. You may discover past issues, childhood habits, or deeper subconscious blocks that keep you from making a healthy change and leading to self-sabotaging.

Meditation is an easy, extremely useful, and harmless process. It is the most practical and beneficial way of connecting with and working on your inner self that is necessary to practice along with incorporating the habit of eating healthy and exercising regularly. If you too have been unable to keep at your diet plan, try meditating, taking help from books on the subject, or seeking help and instructions from online classes or practice groups.

In one of their recent studies, USDA concluded after comparing twenty fruits and vegetables with twenty snack items that fruits and vegetables are healthier and cheaper to consume. Unlike packaged, ready-to-eat snack items, fruits and vegetables may require washing, chopping, storing, and preparation, but the benefits are tremendous. Humans, on average, consume about two thousand calories daily, which can be sufficiently met by fruits and vegetables, which can be bought within as little as 2.50 dollars a day. If you aim to lose the extra fat that has accumulated, it is important to pay attention to what you eat regularly, and one of the most effective ways of achieving results is by cutting off processed food from your diet.

Cravings are common to all of us, and that is when we like to snack on these processed food items. In one of their articles, Scientific American claimed that cravings could sometimes be an indication of hormonal imbalance in our bodies. If you are facing a similar issue, you may consider consulting a professional who can assess your blood work to reveal more about the condition of your organs and the hormones. Sometimes vitamin supplements can also help to keep hormonal levels in check, which otherwise can trigger cravings. This does not mean that you have to give up on your favorite hotdog or the french fry or the soda. If you make it a habit to think that every meal is an opportunity to improve your health, then a new pattern gets registered in both your mind and body, which will enable you to find a balance.

Experts suggest that we limit our daily calorie intake to about two hundred calories, double for athletes or people whose jobs require manual labor. When we restrict ourselves to eat a balanced diet within two hundred calories, we will automatically tend to plan our meals. Sticking to a healthy diet also means decreasing the number of carbohydrates we consume. Some may wonder that this may make us feel hungry frequently, but once you start practicing eating healthy, your taste will have evolved, and your body, mind, and organs will slowly learn and get used to this style of better eating.

Intermittent fasting is one of the ways of enhancing weight loss. This means eating a balanced diet within a 6-8 hour window and fasting for the rest of the day. Nutritionists say that it has great health benefits like lowering cholesterol levels, reducing blood sugar levels, suppressing inflammation, and regulating blood pressure. You may initially feel hungry once you start this method, but the body gradually gets used to the pattern. However, this diet is not recommended for very young people and before you adopt this, remember to consult your doctor.

Hypnotherapy

One piece of advice that is most beneficial for people aspiring to lose weight is to keep track of the calorie you take every day and the calories you burn regularly. The equation is simple, it means that if you consume more calories than you are burning out, you will gain weight, but if you are burning the equal or more amount of calories you consume on a day, you will see a transformation in your physique. Most people struggle to shed weight because several factors hold them back from burning out more calories than they are consuming. Some of these factors could be stress, eating to satisfy emotions, eating out of boredom, childhood eating habits, and social expectations.

It can be difficult for people to stick to their diet plan as they may feel restricted, may feel like they are losing out, and sometimes psychological or emotional issues make one oscillate between dieting and overeating. The problem with the majority of the diets these days is that they are not sustainable. Most diets require consuming a very less amount of calories, sometimes as less as six hundred calories when our body requires two thousand to two thousand five hundred calories daily. This results in making one feel drained quickly. Some of the diets also require you to eat a specific kind of food which limits your food options. This, in the first place, causes resistance because you are not permitted to eat whatever you wish to and also can cause a deficiency of nutrients in your body.

Hypnotherapy is a complementary tool to weight loss. Diet plans, exercise, or intermittent fasting helps to be emotionally and psychologically committed to the weight loss plan for a longer duration of time. Hypnotherapy can be beneficial for people practicing intermittent fasting. We cannot say no to food because we feel like it is a way of rewarding ourselves for doing something good, we feel pressured to eat when someone expects us to, or sometimes boredom makes us munch on snacks. We sometimes cannot resist buying food items because they are on sale or cannot say no to food because we think how many people are hungry around the world. Hypnotherapy is effective in dealing with such thoughts and bring about a behavior change.

Hypnotherapy makes us more mindful of what we eat. It can help us plan our meals better and eliminate trigger foods. This process can also help one sleep better and incorporate habits like drinking more water to help with intermittent fasting. Hypnotherapy can be extremely useful for providing people with the resources that are essential to weight loss. Hypnosis can help one set realistic goals which are central to losing weight, and hypnotizing can further enable to reinforce these goals. Ego and willpower may be boosted by hypnotherapy sessions that can encourage one to stick to their diets. A hypnotherapist can use several methods to make the weight loss process easier. One of the most common and effective combinations is intermittent fasting with hypnotherapy.

The most crucial part of dieting is to keep reminding yourself of positive self-affirmations along with adopting diets and positive lifestyle changes. Remember to be wise, confirm with yourself that you are disciplined, and cultivate self-love to control and monitor what you eat.

CHAPTER 6:

Breakfast Recipes

This chapter will explore some breakfast recipes that you can eat and start your day with.

Green Smoothie

Total Time: 10 minutes

Yields: 2

Nutrition Facts: Calories: 148 | Protein: 6g | Carbs: 10g | Fat: 10g | Fiber: 5g

Ingredients:

- A cup of sliced frozen strawberry
- Two cups of baby spinach
- Half cup of avocado chunks (frozen)
- One and a half cups of almond milk (unsweetened)
- Two tbsps. of hemp seeds
- Three drops of Lakanto Monkfruit extract

Method:

1. First, you need to take a clean blender and add all the ingredients required for preparing the green smoothie. You need to blend till it becomes smooth enough.

2. After that, take two glasses and divide the smoothie equally. Consume it immediately.

Note: You may avoid adding Lakanto Monkfruit extract to your smoothie if you do not wish to make it sweeter. Feel free to adjust the drops according to your preference for sweetness.

Hemp Seed Oatmeal

Total Time: 10 minutes

Yields: 2

Nutrition Facts: Calories: 432 | Carbs: 15.2g | Protein: 11.6g | Fat: 39g | Fiber: 10.7g

Ingredients:

- One tbsp. of flaxseed
- A quarter cup each of
    - Chia seeds
    - Hemp Heart seeds
- One cup of coconut milk or almond milk
- Two tbsps. of erythritol

Method:

1. Take a small-sized saucepan and place every single ingredient into it. Keep the saucepan on top of your oven and set medium heat. You need to keep stirring till you get to see a properly blended mixture.

2. Heat it gently for approximately three to five minutes.

3. After you are done with this part, if you notice that the mixture has turned out to be very stiff, simply add almond milk and that too in a very small quantity.

4. You may serve this dish immediately.

Peach Berry Smoothie

Total Time: 5 minutes

Yields: 1

Nutrition Facts: Calories: 351.3 | Carbs: 61.6g | Protein: 2.7g | Fat: 12.4g | Fiber: 4.5g

Ingredients:

- One cup full of frozen peaches
- Half cup of Greek yogurt
- A quarter cup of coconut milk
- Half tsp. of almond flavoring

Method:

1. Take one blender of high speed and pour the entire quantity of frozen peaches and almond flavoring into it. Let it blend or mix well.

2. After that, you need to check the thickness of the smoothie so that you can adjust it accordingly. If you want your peach berry smoothie to be thinner, then you need to add in more milk. But, if your preference is to enjoy a thicker one, you better add more peaches. Pour it into a medium-sized bowl.

3. Before serving, top it with attractive and tasty toppings such as berries, slivered almonds, and chia seeds.

4. Lastly, enjoy the creamy, sweet bowl of smoothies so that your day starts in the perfect healthy manner.

Avocado Toasts With Poached Eggs

Total Time: 15 minutes

Yields: 4

Nutrition Facts: Calories: 439.8 | Carbs: 26.6g | Protein: 16.2g | Fat: 31.2g | Fiber: 7.5g

Ingredients:

- Two ripe avocados
- Four thick slices of bread
- Two tsps. of lemon juice/ juice of one lime
- Four eggs
- One cup of cheese (grated, gruyere, edam, or any other present on hand)
- Four tsps. of butter (to spread on toast)
- Black pepper (freshly ground)
- Salt (as required)

Method:

1. At first, you need to poach the eggs with the help of your favorite process.

2. In the meantime, slice the ripe avocados in equal halves, as well as take out the stones.

3. After that, take a clean spoon of large size for scooping out its flesh. As you are done with the scooping part, keep the flesh of the avocado into one bowl. Now, it is time to add the lime or lemon juice as well as the required quantity of ground black pepper and salt.

4. The next step is to use a fork for mashing all the ingredients roughly that are inside the bowl.

5. Once you finish mashing, toast the slices of bread—spread butter on top of each slice.

6. Now, you need to take a sufficient amount of avocado mix to spread it onto every single buttered toast slice. Top each slice with one poached egg.

7. For additional taste, sprinkle grated cheese over the poached eggs. Serve it immediately.

Note: For enhancing the taste, you may include either grilled or fresh tomato halves beside the avocado toasts.

Almond Vanilla Granola

Total Time: 2 hours 10 minutes

Yields: 12

Nutrition Facts: Calories: 187.1 | Carbs: 25.3g | Protein: 3.9g | Fat: 8g | Fiber: 2.9g

Ingredients:

- Half cup each of
    - Cane sugar (natural)
    - Water
    - Sliced almonds
- Three and a half cups of oats (old fashioned)
- A quarter cup of grapeseed oil or a quarter cup of canola oil (organic)
- A quarter tsp. of salt
- One tbsp. of vanilla extract

Method:

1. For heating, your oven set the temperature to exactly 200 degrees. Use parchment paper for lining one rimmed cookie sheet of large size.

2. Now, take one large bowl and place the almonds and oats into it. Mix both the ingredients together.

3. Pour salt and cane sugar along with water into one small saucepan and put it over almost medium heat. Keep stirring. The stirring should be continued till the sugar gets dissolved completely. Remove the saucepan from heat. Next, pour in and stir vanilla and canola oil. You also need to pour the almond and oats mixture into the same saucepan. You need to check whether all the ingredients have been thoroughly combined or not; stirring is necessary till then.

4. After that, spread the combined mixture properly on the already lined cookie sheet. Put it inside the preheated oven and bake it for almost two hours. Or, the baking needs to be done until it is super dry for touching. You must not stir at all in this stage. Then the sheet needs to be removed from the oven. Allow it to cool completely, and only then will you be able to break it into chunks. Lastly, store the chunks in a container (air-tight).

Banana Strawberry Overnight Oats

Total time: 5 minutes

Yields: 2

Nutrition Facts: Calories: 326 | Carbs: 63g | Protein: 8g | Fat: 1g | Fiber: 7g

Ingredients:

- One and a half cups of milk (as per your choice)
- One cup of oats (old fashioned)
- A quarter cup of yogurt (strawberry flavored or plain)
- Two tbsps. of honey
- One chopped banana
- Half cup of chopped strawberries

Method:

1. First of all, take a bowl and put the oats in it. Keep it aside.
2. Now, take another bowl of medium size for whisking yogurt, milk, and honey together.
3. Once you are done whisking, pour the wet ingredients into the bowl of oats. Stirring is required for appropriately combining everything.
4. Lastly, the bananas and strawberries must be added and stirred.
5. The bowl is to be kept inside your refrigerator overnight. You may also try out an alternate option by distributing the combined mixture into one mason jar or cup before placing it inside the refrigerator. Enjoy!

Note: In case you want to have a sweeter banana strawberry overnight oat, use either vanilla or strawberry yogurt. For those who do not want it to be sweet, simply use plain yogurt.

Bacon and Avocado Eggs

Total time: 60-65 minutes

Yields: 2

Nutrition Facts: Calories: 407 | Carbs: 2g | Protein: 25g | Fat: 31g | Fiber: 2.3g

Ingredients:

- Four large-sized eggs
- One tsp. of olive oil
- Two and a half ounces of bacon
- Three and a half ounces of avocado
- Pepper and salt

Method:

1. At first, the oven needs to be preheated by setting the temperature to 350 degrees. You may use aluminum foil or parchment paper for lining one baking sheet (rimmed). After lining the sheet, spread the strips of bacon on it. Keep it aside.

2. Take one saucepan and place all the eggs in it and then fill it up with almost cold water. The level of water must be at least an inch above the eggs. Cover the saucepan with a lid and let it boil lightly by setting the flame to high heat. Remove the saucepan from your burner as soon as it begins to boil properly. Keep the pan covered for about fifteen minutes so that the eggs rest inside it. After that, pour ice-cold water into a bowl and place all the eggs in it with the help of one slotted spoon. Let the eggs stay in this manner for five to ten minutes. You may also try another option- keep the boiled eggs in one colander and place it under running cold water till the eggs cool completely. Peel them and keep them aside.

3. Now, it is time to set the already lined baking sheet on your oven's middle rack for cooking the bacon for almost ten to

twenty minutes. It is better to cook till the bacon becomes crispy, and the time may vary as it entirely depends upon the bacon's thickness. Once done, use paper towels for draining slices of bacon. For forming the sails, the cooled bacon needs to be cut into medium-sized triangles.

4. Then, slice the boiled eggs lengthwise. Use a spoon to take out the egg yolks. Place the scooped yolks, olive oil, and avocado in one small-sized bowl. Use a fork for mashing the ingredients of the bowl until combined. For enhancing the taste, you may season with pepper and salt.

5. Lastly comes the assembling part. Spoon the yolk and avocado mixture into the sliced egg whites very generously. Place the sails of bacon in the mixture's center. Serve and enjoy!

High Protein Breakfast Bowl

Total time: 5 minutes

Yields: 1

Nutrition Facts: Calories: 373 | Carbs: 5g | Protein: 33g | Fat: 24g | Fiber: 5g

Ingredients:

- Three and a half ounces of cured salmon or smoked salmon
- Two large-sized boiled eggs (cut them in halves)
- Two tbsps. of cream cheese
- Three ounces of cucumber (ribboned or diced)
- A quarter lemon (cut in chunks, optional)
- Half tsp. of dried chives or bagel seasoning (optional)

Method:

1. Take a bowl of large size and place every single ingredient into it.
2. For adding extra flavor, sprinkle the required quantity of bagel seasoning. If you do not want to add bagel seasoning, then add pepper and salt.
3. Serve.

Note: In case you do not prefer salmon, you may use canned ham, deli turkey, or tuna as a substitute.

Green Omelet

Total time: 20-25 minutes

Yields: 1

Nutrition Facts: Calories: 468 | Carbs: 4g | Protein: 21g | Fat: 41g | Fiber: 2g

Ingredients:

- Two tbsps. of fresh cilantro (finely chopped), or parsley (flat-leaf)
- Two large-sized eggs
- One green chili (finely sliced, seeded)
- Two tbsps. of whipping cream (heavy)
- Four tbsps. of cheddar cheese (shredded)
- One tbsp. of butter
- One and a quarter ounces or a cup of baby spinach or watercress (chopped roughly)
- Pepper and salt (for seasoning)

Method:

1. Take a bowl and pour the eggs into it after cracking them. Add heavy cream, green chili, and cilantro to the bowl. Use a fork for whisking all the ingredients together till the mixture combines well. Next, you need to do the seasoning with an ample quantity of pepper as well as salt as per your taste. Keep the bowl aside.

2. Now, it is time to melt one tbsp. of butter. For that, you will need a small-sized and non-stick pan. Set the flame to medium heat and place the frying pan over the burner. After melting the butter, add in the already prepared egg mixture. You have to move the eggs while it gets cooked with the help of a spatula. Do it for nearly one minute. As soon as you

notice that the exterior edges are becoming opaque, start moving the spatula all around the pan's rim. It helps in loosening the edges. In order to be sure whether the omelet is sliding or not, just shake your frying pan gently.

3. After that, all you need to do is sprinkle shredded cheese on top of the whole omelet and then the watercress. Decrease the heat and cover the pan with a lid. Leave it in this state for a few minutes. Serve after transferring the green omelet to a dish.

Note: For avoiding the spicy nature of green chili, feel free to adjust the taste by including a small lump of yogurt (thick).

Taco Breakfast Skillet

Total Time: 1 hour

Yields: 6

Nutrition facts: Calories: 563 | Carbs: 9g | Protein: 32g | Fat: 44g | Fiber: 4g

Ingredients:

- Ten large-sized eggs
- One pound of ground beef
- Two-thirds cup of water
- Four tbsps. of Taco seasoning
- A quarter cup each of
  - Heavy cream
  - Salsa
  - Sour cream
  - Black olives (sliced)
- One and a half cups of cheddar cheese (shredded, divided)

- One medium-sized peeled avocado (cubed and pitted)
- One diced Roma tomato
- Two sliced green onions
- One sliced jalapeno (optional)
- Two tbsps. of fresh cilantro (torn, optional)

Method:

1. In the beginning, take one skillet of large size and place ground beef in it. Let the beef turn brown over medium to high heat. Drain away the extra fat.

2. Stir in water and taco seasoning to the hot skillet. Lower the heat and allow it to simmer for almost five minutes till the sauce thickens and layers the meat completely. Then, keep aside about half a portion of the beef by taking it out from the large skillet.

3. Now, take one large-sized mixing bowl for whisking the eggs after cracking them. Add a cup of cheese, heavy cream, and whisk for combining perfectly.

4. For preheating the oven, set the temperature to approximately 375 degrees.

5. In the meantime, pour the already prepared egg mixture on top of the remaining meat present in the skillet. Stir with a spatula for combining the eggs and meat. Next, you need to bake for half an hour or till it has become fluffy.

6. After the baking part is over, top it with a half cup of cheese, half portion of seasoned beef, avocado, green onion, olives, tomato, salsa, and sour cream.

7. Before serving, garnish the dish with cilantro and jalapeno.

Low Carb Muesli

Total Time: 9 minutes

Yields: 15

Nutrition Facts: Calories: 217 | Carbs: 6g | Protein: 8g | Fat: 19g | Fiber: 3g

Ingredients:

- One cup each of
  - Sliced almonds
  - Pumpkin seeds
  - Flaked coconut (unsweetened)
  - Sunflower seeds
- Two tsps. of cinnamon
- Half cup each of
  - Hemp hearts
  - Pecans
- A quarter tsp. of stevia drops (vanilla)
- Half tsp. of vanilla extract

Method:

1. First of all, you need to take one large-sized bowl. Pour every single ingredient into the bowl and stir by using a spatula. Stirring helps combine all the ingredients properly.

2. Next, you need to take one baking pan (rimmed) and place the mixed ingredients in it. In the meantime, set the temperature of your oven to 350 degrees. Insert the pan and bake for nearly eight minutes.

3. Once the baking is done, let it cool. You may store it in any container (air-tight).

4. One serving is almost one-third cup, and the taste enhances if almond milk is added to it.

CHAPTER 7:

Lunch Recipes

Are you ready to explore some delicious yet healthy lunch recipes?

Fresh Spinach Frittata

Total Time: 45 minutes

Yields: 4

Nutrition Facts: Calories: 695 | Carbs: 5g | Protein: 34g | Fat: 60g | Fiber: 2g

Ingredients:

- Two tablespoons of butter
- Eight eggs
- One and forth cups of cheddar cheese, shredded
- Salt and pepper
- Chorizo or diced bacon (five-ounce of diced bacon)
- Seven and a half cups of fresh spinach (eight-ounce of fresh spinach)
- One full cup of a heavy whipping cream

Method:

1. At first, you need to set the temperature of the oven to 350 degrees Fahrenheit and preheat.

2. Next, you need to grease a baking dish of about nine by nine or use individual ramekins.

3. In the next step, you need to fry the bacon in the butter, keeping the heat medium. Fry until it is crispy. When the

bacon has become crispy, go on to add the fresh spinach and stir it well until it has wilted.

4. Now take the pan off the heat and let it cool down.

5. Take the eggs and whisk them really well with the fresh cream. When you are done whisking them well, pour them into the dish you are using for baking or in the ramekins.

6. After this, keep adding the spinach, cheese, and bacon on top of it. Bake this for twenty-five minutes to half an hour. Bake it till it is completely st in the middle and has gotten a nice golden color on top.

Notes: What will absolutely make this dish go on another level is if you serve some shredded cabbage and greens on the side along with some homemade dressing. Enjoy!

Thai Curry Soup

Total Time: 22 minutes

Yields: 6

Nutrition Facts: Calories: 323 | Carbs: 7g | Protein: 15g | Fat: 27g | Fiber: 1g

Ingredients:

Things you need for the soup

- 14.5 ounces of full-fat coconut milk
- Two teaspoons of fish sauce
- One teaspoon of honey or any other average nectar
- Four cloves of crushed garlic
- Four properly boneless and skinless chicken thighs
- Two full teaspoons of yellow Thai curry paste
- Three teaspoons of soy sauce

- One full teaspoon of honey or agave nectar
- Two finely chopped green scallion
- Two-inch of minced ginger. Chop them well.

Things you need to add to the soup after it is cooked

- Half a cup of cherry tomatoes sliced in two.
- Three finely chopped green scallions
- Juice of one lime
- One can of straw mushrooms
- One-fourth cup of chopped cilantro

Method:

For the pot,

1. Take all the ingredients for the main soup and then put them in an instant pot and seal it.
2. You need to cook the soup for about twelve minutes under pressure.
3. Release the pressure quickly and take the chicken out. Shred the chicken well and put the chicken back in the soup.
4. Now take all the veggies and add them to the broth, which is hot. Keep the veggies in the broth for some time, scalding them a little. Keep in mind to not overcook them into a mush.

For the slow cooker,

1. When you are using a slow cooker, place all the main ingredients in the cooker and cook them on low heat for about eight hours. And if you are using high heat, it should take about four hours to get cooked properly.
2. Take the veggies and put them in the cooker in the last half an hour. Keep in mind to not overcook the veggies in a mush. Just give them a little scalding so that their freshness is maintained.

3. Take out the chicken from the soup and shred it well. Then put them back in the soup.

For the stove,

1. Take a pot that has a very thick bottom and then place all the soup ingredients and the chicken in it. Cook them well till the chicken has been cooked well and the broth has become flavorful.

2. Take the chicken out and shred it properly. After you have shredded it well, place it back in the soup.

3. Take the veggies and add them to the broth that is cooking. Do not cook the veggies in mush. Give them a little scalding so that you can taste the freshness of the vegetables and the herbs.

Note: *You can always substitute the heavy whipping cream with coconut milk if you want. Thai curry is also available in all the Asian stores near you. You can buy that and then cook it at home.*

Beef Barbacoa

Total Time: 4 hours and 10 minutes

Yields: 9

Nutrition Facts: Calories: 242 | Carbs: 2g | Protein: 32g | Fat: 11g | Fiber: 1g

Ingredients:

- Half a cup of beef broth (you can also use chicken broth if you want)

- Five cloves of minced garlic

- Two tablespoons of fresh lime juice

- Two teaspoons of cumin

- One teaspoon of black pepper

- Two whole bay leaf
- Three beef brisket, or you can also use chuck roast. (trim them and cut them into two-inch chunks)
- Two medium-sized chipotle chiles in adobo. (take the sauce also, about four teaspoons)
- Two tablespoons of apple cider vinegar
- One tablespoon of dried oregano
- Two teaspoons of sea salt
- Half a teaspoon of ground cloves

Methods:

1. Take all the other ingredients except the bay leaf and the beef. Combine the chipotle chiles in adobo sauce, garlic, lime juice, cumin, black pepper, apple cider vinegar, dried oregano, sea salt, ground cloves, along with the broth in a blender. Blend them well till it becomes a smooth puree.

2. Take a slow cooker and, at first, place all the beef chunks in it; after that, pour the puree on top of it. Then, add the two whole bay leaves.

3. If you want to cook it on low heat, it will take about eight to ten hours. And similarly, if you want to cook it over high flame, it will take about four to six hours to be prepared completely. The beef should be fall-apart tender.

4. After that, remove the bay leaves.

5. Take two forks and shred the meat well and stir it for some time in the broth.

6. Cover the container and let it rest for five to ten minutes. This will help the beef take in more flavor.

7. Finally, use the slotted spoon to serve.

Notes: You can use a variety of meat for this recipe, but for perfect Mexican barbacoa, brisket or chuck roast is the best.

Smoked Salmon and Avocado

Total Time: 5 minutes

Yields: 2

Nutrition Facts: Calories: 548 | Proteins: 25g | Carbs: 4g | Fat: 45g | Fiber: 1g

Ingredients:

- Eight ounces of smoked salmon
- Two avocadoes, that is, fourteen ounces of avocadoes
- Salt and pepper according to taste
- Two tablespoons of mayonnaise

Method:

1. At first, take the avocadoes and split them in half. Remove the pit from inside it and then scoop out the entire avocado with the help of a spoon.
2. Place the avocadoes on a plate and keep them aside.
3. Now, take the salmon and the mayonnaise and add them to the plate.
4. Finally, add salt and pepper according to taste on top of it.

Note: Try to get as fresh salmon as possible as that changes the taste completely and uplifts the dish.

Fried Chicken With Broccoli

Total Time: 20 minutes

Yields: 2

Nutrition Facts: Calories: 484 | Protein: 43g | Carbs: 5g | Fat: 31g | Fiber: 2g

Ingredients:

- Two ounces of butter
- Salt and pepper according to taste
- Nine ounces of broccoli
- Fourteen ounces of chicken thighs (boneless)

Method:

1. Take the broccoli and wash it properly. After you have rinsed them well, trim them.
2. Keep in mind to keep the stems intact and cut them into small pieces.
3. Take a frying pan and heat up the butter in it. Keep in mind that the butter should be enough to fry both the broccoli and the chicken in it.
4. Season the chicken from beforehand.
5. Now take the chicken and fry it in the butter. Fry each side for five minutes over medium heat.
6. Fry the chicken until it is golden brown in color. Make sure it is cooked completely.
7. After the chicken has been fried properly, add some butter and then add the broccoli to the pan.
8. Fry for some more minutes.
9. Pepper and salt should be added as per your taste.
10. Serve when hot and enjoy!

Note: *You can also make this dish with many other vegetables which have a low carbohydrate content, like zucchini or spinach, or asparagus. It completely depends on you as to which vegetable you will use. Also, feel free to add your favorite spices for more flavor, like onion powder. You could also add different herbs and paprika if you want.*

Cauliflower Hash

Total Time: 25 minutes

Yields: 2

Nutrition Facts: Calories: 528 | Protein: 18.3g | Carbs: 7g | Fat: 46.7g | Fiber: 3g

Ingredients:

- Half a teaspoon of garlic powder
- One tbs of olive oil
- Four tbs of butter
- Pepper and salt as per your taste
- Four tablespoons of sour cream
- Three ounces of poblano pepper
- 12 ounces of cauliflower
- Four eggs

Method:

1. In the beginning, measure out all the different ingredients that you need and keep everything else prepared.
2. Take a bowl and start mixing the sour cream and the garlic powder together.
3. Keep aside this mix for later use.

4. Take a food processor and rice the cauliflower. Keep in mind to keep the stems intact.

5. Take the poblano pepper and brush some olive oil on it. Fry this for some time over medium to high heat, and then keep it aside.

6. After this, take a pan and add the butter. When it is heated up, add the cauliflower and let it fry for five to six minutes. Fry till the stems are soft.

7. Then chop the poblano pepper well and add it to the cauliflower. When they have been mixed well, remove them from the an and keep them aside.

8. Take the pan again and take some olive oil in it. When the oil is hot, take the eggs and fry them sunny side up.

9. You can also fry the eggs any way you like them.

10. Serve the freshly fried eggs with the cauliflower hash that you just prepared, along with the sour cream dip.

11. Serve with sprinkling some salt and pepper on top.

Note: *The amount of ingredients that has been mentioned is fit for two servings of cauliflower hash with fried eggs.*

Seared Salmon

Total Time: 40 minutes

Yields: 2

Nutrition Facts: Calories: 976 | Protein: 56g | Carbs: 7g | Fat: 80g | Fiber: 3g

Ingredients:

For the lemon sauce and salmon

- Two-thirds cup of heavy whipping cream
- Two tablespoons of fresh parsley (chop them finely)
- Juice of half a lemon
- Half teaspoon of salt
- Two tablespoons of olive oil are needed for searing
- Salt and pepper as per your taste
- Half a cup of a vegetable stalk
- One tablespoon of chives, finely chopped
- One pinch of black pepper
- Boneless fillets of salmon about 1\2" (1.2 centimeters) thick.

For serving

- Fifteen cups of fresh spinach
- Salt and pepper as per taste
- One tablespoon of butter

Method:

For the lemon sauce,

1. Take a small saucepan and then pour all the vegetables in it.
2. Over a high flame, let the vegetables boil for some time.

3. Then let it boil for some time till the stalk is reduced.

4. Then add the lemon, chives, parsley, salt, and pepper to the stalk. Whisk it for some time.

5. Reduce the heat and keep it at a low temperature. Do not cover the pan and keep whisking occasionally.

6. Let this salt get more thickened as you prepare the salmon.

For the salmon,

1. Take a large skillet or a non-stick pan.

2. Over medium to high flame heat some olive oil in it.

3. Take the pepper and the salt and season the fish on both the sides, then place it on the pan, making sure the skin side is facing down.

4. Let it sear for about four minutes till the fish is brown and crispy.

5. You need to flip the fish now; keep in mind to reduce the flame before that so that the fish does not get burnt. Cook for another three to five minutes until the fish turns golden and crispy on the outside and a light shade of pink on the inside.

6. Take a serving plate and place the fish on it. Serve hot!

For serving,

1. Take a large frying pan and add the butter. Let it melt completely over medium heat.

2. You need to add the spinach now while keeping the flame medium-high.

3. Take tongs and toss the spinach for some time in the butter. Toss it till the spinach gets wilted.

4. Add the pepper and the salt according to your taste, and remove the spinach from the pan.

5. When you are serving, make sure to squeeze some lemon juice over the salmon and serve with the sauteed spinach on the side.

Note: Before using the salmon, let it rest for about fifteen minutes and make sure it is at room temperature. This helps the salmon to get cooked evenly. You can store the cooked salmon in your fridge for about three days. You can store the sauce in an air-tight container in your fridge for about three days. You will need to heat up the sauce well before using it every time.

Arugula and Cauliflower Shrimp

Total time: 30 minutes

Yields: 4

Nutrition Facts: Calories:308 | Protien: 24g | Carbs: 13g | Fat: 18g | Fiber: 5g

Ingredients:

For the shrimp

- One tablespoon of paprika
- Half a teaspoon of cayenne pepper
- Freshly ground black pepper and salt
- One pound shrimp (peeled and deveined)
- Two teaspoons of garlic powder
- One tablespoon of extra-virgin olive oil

For the cauliflower grits

- Four cups of riced cauliflower
- Half a cup of goat cheese (crumbled)
- Freshly ground black pepper and salt
- One tablespoon of unsalted butter

- One cup of whole milk

For the garlic arugula

- Three very thinly sliced garlic cloves
- Freshly ground black pepper and salt as per taste
- One tablespoon of extra-virgin olive oil
- Four cups of baby arugula

Method:

For the spicy shrimp,

1. Take a large zip-top plastic bag and place the shrimp in that.
2. In a bowl take the garlic powder and the paprika and mix them nicely in it. Add the cayenne to it and mix it well.
3. Pour this mixture into the bag of shrimp and toss the bag really well. Toss the bag really well till all the shrimp are nicely covered with this paste.
4. Keep this bag of shrimp on the fridge for some time till you prepare the grits.

For the cauliflower grits,

1. Take a pot and over a medium heat melt the butter in it. Now add the cauliflower rice in it and cook for two minutes till it releases moisture.
2. Take half of the milk and stir it well, bringing it to shimmer. Simmer it for some time till the cauliflower absorbs some of the milk.
3. Now add the remaining milk and make it simmer till it becomes a thick creamy paste, for about ten minutes.
4. Add the cheese in it and add the salt and pepper to it.

For the garlic arugula,

1. Take a frying pan or a big skillet and heat olive oil in it. Over a medium heat, sautee the garlic in it for a minute.

2. After that, take the arugula and stir it in the olive oil for three minutes. Give salt and pepper as per taste.

3. Serve this by diving the grits among four plates and place a quarter of arugula on top and a quarter of shrimp.

Note: The fresh the ingredients are, the tastier the dish will be. So, make sure to choose only the freshest of the ingredients you get.

CHAPTER 8:

Dinner Recipes

Let us now explore some sumptuous dinner recipes for your intermittent fasting diet plan.

Fried Cauliflower Rice With Chicken

Total time: 35 minutes

Yields: 4

Nutrition Facts: Calories: 427 | Carbs: 25g | Protein: 45g | Fat: 16g | Fiber: 7g

Ingredients:

- Four large-sized eggs (beaten)
- One and a half lb. of skinless, boneless chicken breast (crushed to uniform thickness)
- Two small-sized carrots (chopped finely)
- Two bell peppers (red, finely chopped)
- Two finely chopped cloves of garlic
- One onion (chopped finely)
- Half cup of thawed, frozen peas
- Four cups of cauliflower rice
- Four finely chopped scallions
- Two tbsps. each of
    - Soy sauce (low-sodium)
    - Grapeseed oil

- Two tsps. of rice vinegar
- Pepper and Kosher salt

Method:

1. Take one deep and large-sized skillet and set the heat to medium temperature. Pour one tbsp. of oil and heat it. Once the oil becomes hot enough, add the entire quantity of chicken. Cook each side for three to four minutes till the color turns golden brown. Now, you need to transfer the cooked or fried chicken to your cutting board. Before you start slicing the chicken, allow it to rest for about five to six minutes. Pour one tbsp. of oil into the skillet and add the beaten eggs for scrambling. You might need one to two minutes to cook the scrambled eggs. Transfer it to a small-sized bowl.

2. Now, you need to add carrot, onion, and bell pepper to the same skillet and cook for nearly four to five minutes. You need to stir all the ingredients quite often till all of them become tender. As soon as you get to see the tender texture, stir in the finely chopped garlic cloves and cook for one more minute. It is time to toss with thawed peas and scallions.

3. After that, add soy sauce, rice vinegar, cauliflower, pepper, and salt, and tossing is required for combining all the ingredients properly. Do not stir for two to three minutes so that the cauliflower begins to get the brown color and also gets the time to sit. Lastly, you need to toss with scrambled eggs and sliced chicken.

Turkey Tacos

Total Time: 25 minutes

Yields: 4

Nutrition Facts: Calories: 472 | Carbs: 30g | Protein: 28g | Fat: 27g | Fiber: 6g

Ingredients:

- One lb. of ground turkey (extra-lean)
- One small-sized chopped red onion
- Two tsps. of oil
- One finely chopped clove of garlic
- One sliced avocado
- Eight corn tortillas (whole-grain, warmed)
- One tbsp. of taco seasoning (sodium-free)
- A quarter cup of sour cream
- One cup of chopped lettuce
- Half cup of Mexican cheese (shredded)
- Salsa (required for serving)

Method:

1. First of all, you need to take one large-sized skillet and pour oil into it. Heat the poured oil over medium to high flame. Next, you have to add the chopped onion and stir for about five to six minutes until tender. Once the onion becomes tender, add in the chopped garlic. Stir and cook for a minute.

2. Now, you need to add one lb. of turkey and use a spoon to break it evenly. Cook for almost five minutes until the turkey becomes nearly brown. Then, you have to add a cup of water and taco seasoning. Let it simmer for about six to seven minutes until it gets decreased to almost half portion.

3. Next, it is time to fill in the tortillas with cooked turkey. Top with cheese, salsa, avocado, sour cream, and lettuce.

Sheet Pan Steak

Total Time: 50 minutes

Yields: 4

Nutrition Facts: Calories: 464 | Carbs: 26g | Protein: 42g | Fat: 22g | Fiber: 8g

Ingredients:

- One a quarter lb. of bunch broccolini (trimmed into lengths of 2 inches)
- Four finely chopped garlic cloves
- One lb. of small-sized cremini mushrooms (halved and trimmed)
- Three tbsps. of olive oil
- One 15 ounce can of cannellini beans (low-sodium and rinsed)
- A quarter tsp. of red pepper flakes
- One and a half lb. of steaks of New York strip (excess fat trimmed off)
- Pepper and Kosher salt

Method:

1. At first, the oven needs to be preheated, and for that, you need to set the temperature to exactly 450 degrees. Take one large-sized baking sheet (rimmed) and toss in broccolini, mushrooms, red pepper flakes, oil, garlic, and a quarter tsp. each of pepper and salt. After that, place your baking sheet inside the oven. All the ingredients need to be roasted for approximately fifteen minutes.

2. Next, you have to make the necessary space required for placing the steaks. For that, it is better to push the roasted mixture towards the pan's edges. Before placing the steaks in the middle of your pan, season with a quarter tsp. each of pepper and Kosher salt. Now, it is time to roast the seasoned steaks, and each side must be roasted for five to seven minutes. Roast according to your desired doneness. Then, you have to take out the roasted steaks and place them on a clean cutting board. Slice only after allowing to rest for five minutes.

3. In the meantime, keep the beans on the same baking sheet. Toss the beans for combining evenly—roast for three to four minutes until the beans are heated thoroughly. Lastly, enjoy the dish by serving vegetables and roasted beans with steak.

Spaghetti Bolognese

Total Time: One and a half hours

Yields: 4

Nutrition Facts: Calories: 450 | Carbs: 31g | Protein: 32g | Fat: 23g | Fiber: 6g

Ingredients:

- One and a quarter lb. of ground turkey
- One large-sized spaghetti squash
- Half tsp. of garlic powder
- Three tbsps. of olive oil
- One small-sized finely chopped onion
- Four finely chopped garlic cloves
- Three cups or two 15-ounce cans of diced tomatoes (fresh)
- Eight ounces of small-sized and sliced cremini mushrooms

- Basil (freshly chopped)
- One 8 ounce can of tomato sauce (sugarless and low-sodium)
- Pepper and Kosher salt

Method:

1. First of all, you need to preheat your oven by setting the temperature to exactly 400 degrees. Meanwhile, halve the large-sized spaghetti squash lengthwise and also discard the seeds. After that, rub every single half with half tbsp. of oil as well as season the halves with a quarter tsp. each of pepper and salt along with garlic powder. Take a baking sheet (rimmed) and place the seasoned spaghetti squash on it with the skin side upwards. Let it roast for more than half an hour, say about forty minutes or until tender. Once the roasting is done, allow cooling for the next ten minutes.

2. In the meantime, take one skillet of large size and heat two tbsps. of oil over medium heat. As soon as the oil becomes hot, add the finely chopped onion in it after seasoning with a quarter tsp. each of pepper and salt. Stir occasionally and cook for about six minutes until the onions become tender. Next, you need to add in the turkey and use a spoon to break it into very small pieces. Cook until it turns brown, or for seven minutes. After this, you also need to add in chopped garlic cloves and stir for a minute.

3. Now, you have to set aside the already prepared turkey mixture to a side and place the cremini mushrooms on the other side of the pan. Stir occasionally and cook for almost five minutes so that the mushrooms become perfectly tender. Now, mix it with the turkey and add tomato sauce and tomatoes into it. Let it simmer for approximately ten minutes.

4. When you observe the sauce simmering, you have to transfer the squash to plates after scooping it out. Pour the Turkey Bolognese on top. If you feel like it, you may sprinkle basil before serving.

Pork Tenderloin With Brussels Sprouts and Butternut Squash

Total Time: 50 minutes

Yields: 4

Nutrition Facts: Calories: 401 | Carbs: 25g | Protein: 44g | Fat: 15g | Fiber: 6g

Ingredients:

- One and three-fourth lb. of trimmed pork tenderloin
- Three tbsps. of canola oil
- Two peeled cloves of garlic
- Two sprigs of fresh thyme
- Four cups each of
  - Butternut squash (diced)
  - Brussels sprouts (halved and trimmed)
- Pepper
- Salt

Method:

1. In the beginning, all you need to do is preheat your oven by setting the temperature to exactly 400 degrees. While the oven gets preheated, season the pork tenderloin properly with the required amount of pepper and salt. Take one large-sized pan of cast-iron and pour one tbsp. of oil into it. Heat the oil on medium or high heat. As you get to see that the oil is shimmering, add the seasoned tenderloin and cook for eight to twelve minutes. Sear until the tenderloin turns golden brown on all sides. Then, you need to transfer it to a large-sized plate.

2. Next, you need to add the remaining quantity of canola oil, garlic, and thyme to your pan. Cook the ingredients for almost a minute till you get their aroma. Now, it is time to add butternut squash, brussels sprouts, and one pinch each of pepper and salt. Cook for five to six minutes by occasional stirring till all the veggies attain a slight brown color.

3. Then, you need to keep the cooked tenderloin on top of the vegetables. Transfer all the ingredients to your oven. The roasting must be done till the vegetables become tender or till your meat thermometer registers a temperature of 140 degrees when it is introduced in the tenderloin's thickest part. Roasting might take nearly fifteen to twenty minutes.

4. After that, wear oven gloves for safety and take out the hot pan from your oven very carefully. Before slicing the tenderloin, let it rest for five minutes and then serve with vegetables. You may also toss the veggies with balsamic vinaigrette before serving. Enjoy!

Pork Chops With Bloody Mary Tomato Salad

Total Time: 25 minutes

Yields: 4

Nutrition Facts: Calories: 400 | Carbs: 8g | Protein: 39g | Fat: 23g | Fiber: 3g

Ingredients:

- Two tsps. each of
    - Horseradish (prepared, squeezed dry)
    - Worcestershire sauce
- Two tbsps. each of
    - Red wine vinegar
    - Olive oil

- One pint of halved cherry tomatoes
- Half tsp. each of
  - Celery seeds
  - Tabasco
- Two stalks of celery (thinly sliced)
- A quarter cup of flat-leaf parsley (finely chopped)
- Four small-sized or about two and a quarter lb. of bone-in pork chops (thickness of one inch)
- Half small-sized and thinly sliced red onion
- One small head of lettuce (green-leaf, leaves torn)
- Pepper
- Kosher salt

Method:

1. Before getting ready to prepare the super delicious dish, you need to heat the grill on medium to high heat. Meanwhile, take a large-sized bowl and whisk together vinegar, oil, horseradish, celery seeds, Worcestershire sauce, Tabasco, and a quarter tsp. of salt. After the whisking is over, toss with celery, onion, and cherry tomatoes.

2. Now it is time to use half a teaspoon each of pepper and salt for seasoning pork chops and let it grill. Each side must be grilled for six to seven minutes or till the chops become golden brown and thoroughly cooked.

3. Next, you need to place the leafy parsley inside the tomatoes by folding and serve it over greens and grilled pork. You may enhance the taste by consuming it with mashed potatoes or cauliflower.

Wild Cajun Spicy Salmon

Total Time: 30 minutes

Yields: 4

Nutrition Facts: Calories: 408 | Carbs: 9g | Protein: 42g | Fat: 23g | Fiber: 3g

Ingredients:

- Half lb. of head cauliflower (chopped into florets)
- One and a half lb. of salmon fillets (wild Alaskan)
- One lb. of head broccoli (chopped into florets)
- Four medium-sized diced tomatoes
- Half tsp. of garlic powder
- Three tbsps. of olive oil
- Taco seasoning (sodium-free)

Method:

1. At first, the oven needs to be preheated and for that, set the temperature of your oven to exactly 375 degrees. Keep the fillets of salmon in one baking dish. Next, you need to take one small-sized bowl and combine half a cup of water and taco seasoning in it. Once the mixing is done, pour it over the fillets and let it bake for nearly fifteen minutes or till the salmon becomes opaque throughout.

2. In the meantime, pulse both broccoli and cauliflower by using a food processor until the veggies become evenly chopped as well as riced.

3. Now, take one large-sized skillet and heat olive oil over medium heat. When the oil becomes hot, add in the chopped broccoli and cauliflower and then sprinkle garlic powder. Toss and cook until all the ingredients become tender or for about five to six minutes.

4. Lastly, place the baked salmon fillets on top of the rice. Top with the diced tomatoes and serve.

Sweet Potato and Black Bean Burrito

Total Time: 1 hour 15 minutes

Yields: 8-12

Nutrition facts: Calories: 575.2 | Carbs: 102g | Protein: 19.8g | Fat: 10.3g | Fiber: 15.9g

Ingredients:

- Twelve flour tortillas (10 inches)
- Five cups of peeled sweet potatoes (cubed)
- Three and a half cups of diced onions
- Two tsps. of broth or two tsps. of vegetable oil
- Four pressed or minced garlic cloves
- Four tsps. each of
    - Ground coriander
    - Ground cumin
- One tbsp. of fresh and minced green chili pepper
- Two-third cup of cilantro leaf (lightly packed)
- Four and a half cups or three 15-ounce cans of black beans (drained and cooked)
- Two tbsps. of lemon juice (fresh)
- One tsp. of salt
- Fresh salsa

Method:

1. Preheat your oven and set the temperature to 350 degrees.

2. Take one medium-sized saucepan and keep the sweet potatoes in it along with water and salt to cover.

3. Cover the saucepan and let it boil. Allow the ingredients to simmer for almost ten minutes till the sweet potatoes become tender.

4. Then, you have to drain out the remaining water and keep it aside.

5. After cooking the sweet potatoes, take one medium-sized saucepan or skillet and pour oil into it. After the oil becomes warm, add in garlic, chili, and onions.

6. Cover the pan and let the ingredients cook on low-medium heat. You need to stir occasionally for almost six to seven minutes till the onions become tender.

7. Next, you need to add ground coriander and cumin to the pan. Cook for another two to three minutes, and you must not forget to stir frequently.

8. After that, set your pan aside by removing it from heat.

9. Now, it is time to take out your food processor. You have to combine cilantro, the entire quantity of black beans, salt, already cooked and tender sweet potatoes, and lemon juice in your food processor. Puree all the ingredients till it becomes perfectly smooth. In case you do not have a food processor, you may mash all the ingredients with the help of your hand by placing them in a large-sized bowl.

10. After that, take one large-sized mixing bowl for transferring the mixture of sweet potato. Mix spices and cooked onions in that mixture.

11. When you are done mixing all the ingredients, take one large-sized baking dish and oil it lightly.

12. Place two-third to a three-fourth cup of this filling inside each tortilla. Then, you need to roll the tortillas and place them in the oiled baking dish with the seam side downwards.

13. Cover the dish very tightly with the help of a foil. Let it bake for half an hour.

14. Top it with fresh salsa. Your dish is ready to be served.

CHAPTER 9:

Snacks & Dessert Recipes

Here are some tasty and easy snacks and desserts for your intermittent fasting regime.

Tortilla Chips

Total Time: 35 minutes

Yields: 4-6

Nutrition facts: Calories: 140 | Carbs: 21g | Protein: 1g | Fat: 7g | Fiber: 3g

Ingredients:

- One cup of almond flour
- Two cups of shredded mozzarella
- Half tsp. of chili powder
- One tsp. each of
    - Garlic powder
    - Kosher salt
- Black pepper (freshly ground)

Method:

1. First of all, preheating your oven is necessary and for that, set the temperature of your oven to exactly 35o degrees. Take two large-sized baking sheets and line them by using parchment paper.

2. After that, take one bowl (microwave safe) and use it for melting mozzarella. This might need almost a minute and thirty seconds. Then, add garlic powder, almond flour, chili

powder, salt, and black pepper. You have to use your hands at this stage for kneading dough. Make sure that a soft ball is formed.

3. Once you are done kneading the dough, place it in between both the parchment paper sheets. Then, give it a rectangle shape with a thickness of one-eighth inch. Take one pizza cutter or sharp knife for cutting the dough into small triangles.

4. Next, you have to spread out the chips on the baking sheets that are already prepared and let them bake. The baking must be done for almost twelve to fifteen minutes till it begins to crisp and the edges become golden in color.

Avocado Chips

Total Time: 40 minutes

Yields: 15

Nutrition facts: Calories: 120 | Carbs: 4g | Protein: 7g | Fat: 10g | Fiber: 2g

Ingredients:

- Three-forth cup of Parmesan (freshly grated)
- One large-sized ripe avocado
- Half tsp. each of
    - Italian seasoning
    - Garlic powder
- One tsp. of lemon juice
- Black pepper (freshly ground)
- Kosher salt

Method:

1. In the beginning, preheat your oven by setting the temperature to 325 degrees. Take two baking sheets and use parchment paper for lining both of them. Now, take one medium-sized bowl and a fork for mashing avocado until smooth. As you are done with the mashing part, stir in lemon juice, Parmesan, Italian seasoning, and garlic powder. You need to do the seasoning with pepper and salt.

2. Scoop teaspoon size heaps of the prepared mixture on the lined baking sheet. You need to make sure that there is a gap of three inches between each scoop. Next, take a measuring cup or spoon and use its backside for flattening each scoop having a width of three inches. Place the baking sheet inside the oven and allow it to bake for half an hour until golden and crisp. Take out the sheet from the oven and let it cool completely. Satisfy your taste buds by serving at usual room temperature.

Burger Fat Bombs

Total Time: 30 minutes

Yields: 20

Nutrition facts: Calories: 80 | Carbs: 0g | Protein: 5g | Fat: 7g | Fiber: 0g

Ingredients:

- One lb. of ground beef
- Two tbsps. of cold butter (trimmed into twenty pieces)
- Half tsp. of garlic powder
- Two ounces of cheddar (trimmed into twenty pieces)
- Tomatoes (thinly sliced, for serving)
- Lettuce leaves (fresh, for serving)

- Mustard (needed for serving)
- Cooking spray
- Black pepper (freshly ground)
- Kosher salt

Method:

1. At first, your oven needs to be preheated at a temperature of 375 degrees. Use the required quantity of cooking spray for greasing a very small muffin tin. Then, take one medium-sized bowl and, in it, season ground beef with salt, pepper, and garlic powder.

2. Next, you need to place one tsp. of beef into each cup of the muffin tin and press it in such a manner so that it covers the bottom completely. Keep one piece of cold butter on it, and again press one tsp. of beef so that the butter gets covered completely.

3. After that, you have to transfer one piece of cheddar into each muffin cup. Press the remaining amount of beef softly over the cheese.

4. Now, it is time for baking. Bake for about fifteen minutes and check that the meat is thoroughly cooked. Allow it to cool slightly.

5. Lastly, take one spatula (metal offset) and use it for releasing every single burger from your muffin tin. It is better to serve with mustard, tomatoes, and lettuce leaves.

Ice-cream

Total Time: 8 hours 15 minutes

Yields: 8

Nutrition Facts: Calories: 279 | Carbs: 36g | Protein: 3.3g | Fat: 15g | Fiber: 2g

Ingredients:

- Two cups of heavy cream
- Two 15-ounce cans of coconut milk
- One tsp. of vanilla extract (pure)
- A quarter cup of sweetener
- A pinch of Kosher salt

Method:

1. Before you start preparing this mouth-watering ice cream, you have to keep the coconut milk inside the refrigerator for a minimum time of three hours or, ideally, overnight.

2. For making whipped coconut, you need to take one large-sized bowl and spoon out coconut cream in it and leave the liquid inside the can. After that, take one hand mixer and use it for beating coconut cream till it becomes very creamy. Keep it aside.

3. The next step is to prepare the whipped cream. For that, take one separate large-sized bowl and hand mixer. Beat the heavy cream in it till you get to see the formation of very soft peaks. Then, beat in vanilla and sweetener.

4. Your next step is to fold the already prepared whipped coconut into the whipped cream. Now, transfer the entire mixture into one loaf pan.

5. Put the pan in your refrigerator and let it freeze for almost five hours until solid.

Jalapeno Egg Cups

Total Time: 45 minutes

Yields: 12

Nutrition Facts: Calories: 190.58 | Carbs: 1.56g | Protein: 12.85g | Fat: 14.4g | Fiber: 0.16g

Ingredients:

- Ten large-sized eggs
- Half cup each of
    - Shredded mozzarella
    - Shredded cheddar
- A quarter cup of sour cream
- Twelve slices of bacon
- One tsp. of garlic powder
- Two jalapenos (one thinly sliced and the other one minced)
- Black pepper (Freshly ground)
- Kosher salt
- Cooking spray (non-stick)

Method:

1. For preheating your oven, set the temperature to exactly 375 degrees. Take one large-sized skillet and cook bacon in it on medium heat. The cooking must be done till the bacon attains a slight brown color and is a bit pliable. Line a plate with a paper towel and keep the cooked bacon on it to drain.

2. In the meantime, take one large-sized bowl and whisk together sour cream, eggs, minced jalapeno, garlic powder, and mozzarella, and cheddar cheese. Season all the ingredients with pepper and salt.

3. Next, you have to grease one muffin tin by using a cooking spray. Once you have finished greasing, line each cup with a bacon slice and then pour in the egg mixture. Top every single cup with one slice of jalapeno.

4. Bake for approximately twenty minutes, and the eggs must not look wet. If it looks wet, then bake for another one or two minutes. Let the egg cups cool slightly, and then remove them from the tin.

Rosemary Crackers

Total Time: 1 hour

Yields: 140

Nutrition Facts: Calories: 27 | Carbs: 4g | Protein: 0.7g | Fat: 0.8g | Fiber: 0.2g

Ingredients:

- Half cup of coconut flour

- Two and a half cups of almond flour

- Half tsp. each of

    - Onion powder

    - Chopped dried rosemary

- One tsp. of flaxseed meal (ground)

- Three large-sized eggs

- One tbsp. of olive oil (Extra-virgin)

- A quarter tsp. of kosher salt

Method:

1. At first, the oven needs to be preheated by setting the temperature to 325 degrees. Meanwhile, take parchment paper for lining one baking sheet. Whisk flax meal, coconut

flour, almond flour, onion powder, rosemary, and salt together in one large bowl. Then, add in oil and eggs and combine all the ingredients evenly. You have to mix it continuously till the dough takes the shape of one large ball.

2. Now, you have to sandwich the dough that you have made in between two parchment pieces of paper and then roll to a thickness of one-fourth inch. After that, use a knife for cutting into squares. Transfer all the squares to the baking sheet that you have prepared in the beginning.

3. Bake for almost fifteen minutes till the crackers attain a golden color. You can store the crackers in any resealable container, but before that, it is necessary to cool them properly.

Bacon Guac Bombs

Total Time: 45 minutes

Yields: 15

Nutrition Facts: Calories: 156 | Carbs: 1.4g | Protein: 3.4g | Fat: 15.2g | Fiber: 1.3g

Ingredients:

- Twelve bacon slices (crumbled and cooked)

For preparing Guacamole

- Six ounces of softened cream cheese
- Two avocados (peeled, pitted, and mashed)
- One clove of garlic (minced)
- One lime juice
- One small-sized jalapeno (chopped)
- A quarter minced red onion
- Half tsp. each of

- Chili powder
- Cumin
- Two tbsps. of cilantro (freshly chopped)
- Black pepper (freshly ground)
- Kosher salt

Method:

1. At first, you need to take one large-sized mixing bowl to combine all the ingredients of guacamole. Keep stirring till the mixture becomes smooth (a few chunks won't cause any problem), and then season with pepper and salt. Transfer the bowl to the refrigerator and keep it inside for half an hour.

2. Now, take one large plate and keep the crumbled bacon on it. Use one small-sized cookie scoop for scooping the already prepared guacamole mixture. Place one scoop of mixture in each bacon and then roll for coating in bacon. Repeat the same process till all the bacon, and the entire quantity of guacamole mixture are used up. Store in your refrigerator.

Chocolate Protein Shake

Total Time: 5 minutes

Yields: 1

Nutrition facts: Calories: 241 | Carbs: 28g | Protein: 26g | Fat: 3g | Fiber: 7g

Ingredients:

- Half cup of ice
- Three-fourth cup of almond milk
- Two tbsps. each of
  - Cocoa powder (unsweetened)
  - Hemp seeds (more may be required for serving)
  - Almond butter
- One tbsp. of chia seeds (more may be needed for serving)
- Half tbsp. of vanilla extract (pure)
- Two-three tbsps. of sugar substitute (keto-friendly)
- A pinch of kosher salt

Method:

1. Pour all the ingredients into a blender for combining appropriately. Keep blending until smooth.
2. After that, pour the protein shake into one large-sized glass.
3. Before serving, garnish with a little bit more hemp seeds and chia seeds. Enjoy!

Chocolate Mousse

Total Time: 10 minutes

Yields: 4

Nutrition facts: Calories: 218 | Carbs: 5g | Protein: 2g | Fat: 23g | Fiber: 2g

Ingredients:

- A quarter cup each of
  - Powdered sweetener
  - Cocoa powder (unsweetened, sifted)
- One cup of whipping cream (heavy)
- One tsp. of vanilla extract
- A quarter tsp. of kosher salt

Method:

1. The very first step of making chocolate mousse is whisking the entire quantity of cream till it becomes thick. For whisking, you may opt for either any hand mixer or stand mixer.
2. Next, you have to add sweetener, cocoa powder, salt, and vanilla extract. Keep whisking till the ingredients are combined smoothly.

Note: Those who are willing to make a bit lighter mousse must whisk the egg whites of three large-sized eggs to firm peaks. Then, it must be folded into your mousse mixture for combining as required.

Brown Butter Pralines

Total Time: 16 minutes

Yields: 10

Nutrition facts: Calories: 338 | Carbs: 3g | Protein: 2g | Fat: 36g | Fiber: 2g

Ingredients:

- Two cups of chopped pecans
- Two sticks of salted butter
- Two-third cups each of
    - Granular sweetener
    - Heavy cream
- Half tsp. of xanthan gum
- Sea salt (as required)

Method:

1. At first, you need to prepare one cookie sheet by using parchment paper. You may also use a baking mat (silicone).

2. Take one saucepan so that you can brown the salted butter in it on medium to high heat. Don't forget to stir often. Next, you need to stir in xanthan gum, sweetener, and heavy cream. Once you are done stirring all these ingredients, remove the pan from heat and keep it aside.

3. Meanwhile, stir in all the chopped pecans and then keep the container in the fridge for almost an hour for firming up. You will get to see that the mixture has thickened. Next, scoop out a total number of ten cookie shapes and place them on the baking sheet that you have already prepared. If you want, you may sprinkle salt. Allow the butter pralines to refrigerate until hardened.

4. Choose any air-tight container for storing and keep the container inside the refrigerator until serving.

CHAPTER 10:

A 21-Day Meal Plan for You to Try

This chapter will provide you a 21-Day meal plan that follows the 16/8 method of intermittent fasting.

Day 1

11 am – Sausage and Egg Breakfast Bowl

Total Time: 7 minutes

Yields: 1

Nutrition Facts: Calories: 340 | Protein: 18g |Carbs: 20g | Fiber: 1g | Fat: 20g

Ingredients:

- One-fourth cup of sausages, which has been cooked and crumbled
- Cheddar cheese needs to be sprinkled
- One tablespoon of butter
- Two whole eggs
- Salt and pepper according to taste

Method:

1. The first step that you need to start making this dish with is by breaking open the two eggs that you have taken into a bowl and then scramble them with a fork until you mix them together well.

2. Add the butter to a skillet for some time over medium-high heat.

3. When the butter is melted, add the eggs to that pan and stir them around well.

4. Make sure to not overcook the eggs in the butter; else, they will taste soggy.

5. When you see that the eggs have been perfectly cooked in the way you like it, add the sausages to the pan and also the cheese.

6. Once you have mixed them well, remove them from the pan.

7. Add salt and pepper according to your taste and serve them hot.

Notes: Make sure you take fresh eggs as that will enhance the taste of the dish even more. Otherwise, the sausages will not be well complimented.

3 pm - Easy Keto Bread

Total Time: 5 minutes

Yields: 1

Nutrition Facts: Calories: 344 | Carbs: 8g | Protein: 22g | Fiber: 3g | Fat: 25g

Ingredients:

- Three tablespoons of almond flour
- One-fourth cup of parmesan cheese that has been shredded. (30 grams)
- Half teaspoon of garlic powder
- Pepper according to taste
- One large egg that has been beaten
- Half a teaspoon of baking powder
- One teaspoon of fresh rosemary that has been finely chopped

- Salt to taste
- Unsalted butter that has been melted

Method:

1. Take a bowl that is microwave-proof.

2. Start taking all the ingredients in it that is the almond flour, parmesan cheese, garlic powder, baking powder, rosemary, salt and pepper, melted unsalted butter, and egg.

3. Stir these ingredients for some time till there are no lumps.

4. Put the bowl in the microwave for 90 seconds until you see that the bread has risen.

5. Let the bowl cool down for some time.

6. Serve and enjoy.

Notes: The baking powder should be added in the perfect amount; otherwise, the bread will either not rise if it is too little, or the mixture will spill out of the bowl if the amount of baking powder is too much.

5 pm – Chicken Stir Fry

Total Time: 55 minutes

Yields: 6

Nutrition Facts: Calories: 240 |Protein: 17g | Carbs: 16g | Fat: 12g | Fiber: 3g

Ingredients:

For the chicken

- One pound of boneless chicken thighs. Remove the skin, cut the chicken into bite-size chunks, and pat them to become completely dry.
- One teaspoon of kosher salt
- One tablespoon of arrowroot flour

- Two tablespoons of avocado oil. Split them into two portions.
- Half a teaspoon of black pepper

For the stir fry

- Half a medium yellow onion that has been sliced thinly
- Two bell peppers that have been julienned
- Two small-sized carrots that have been peeled well and thinly sliced
- Four ounces of water chestnuts that have been drained well
- One teaspoon of red chili pepper flakes
- One big pinch of kosher salt
- Eight ounces of broccoli florets
- Four ounces of sugar snap peas
- One and a half tablespoons of sesame oil

For the sauce

- Six garlic cloves that have been minced
- Two tablespoons of apple cider vinegar
- Half a cup of coconut milk
- One and a half tablespoons of minced ginger

Method:

1. In a bowl mix the chicken thighs that you have with one tbs of oil.
2. After that, add the rest ingredients and mix all of them properly so that the chicken is coated with all the ingredients really well.

3. For about two minutes heat a big saute pan over a medium-high flame. Now take that other tablespoon of oil and heat it in the pan for another minute.

4. When the oil is fully heated, add the chicken in a single layer on the pan and make sure that the chicken is not overcooked.

5. Make sure to cook each side until they are golden brown and crispy.

6. When the chicken is ready, take it out from the pan and keep it aside.

7. Now add the onions to the pan, and to that, add a big pinch of that kosher salt.

8. Cook the onion nicely for about two minutes and keep in mind to stir them occasionally. When the onion is half cooked, add the bell peppers, carrots, broccoli, the sugar snap peas and cook all this for about five to seven minutes.

9. Cover the pan with a lid so that everything is cooked well. Make sure to remove the lid occasionally and stir all the ingredients so that the heat is evenly distributed.

10. When things are looking to be almost cooked, add the water chestnuts to it and continue cooking for some time.

11. Take a bowl and mix all the ingredients well that are needed for the sauce. Now add this sauce to the stir fry that was already cooking. Cook everything for about two to three minutes.

12. Now that the vegetables and the sauce is well cooked take the chicken and add that into the pan. To that, put in the chili pepper and the sesame oil to it.

13. Keep this over the heat for another couple of minutes so that all the flavors are well mixed.

14. Take a quick taste and see whether the seasonings are all according to your taste. Add more if you want.

15. Garnish this with sesame seeds and scallions.

Note: Serve this with brown rice to get the best taste out of it.

Day 2

11 am – Black Bean and Avocado Eggs

Total Time: 10 minutes

Yields: 2

Nutrition Facts: Calories: 356 | Proteins: 20g | Carbs: 18g | Fiber: 11g | Fat: 20g

Ingredients:

- Two tablespoons of rapeseed oil
- One large garlic clove that has been sliced
- Four hundred grams can of black beans
- One-fourth of teaspoons of cumin seeds
- A handful of freshly chopped coriander
- One large red chili that has been deseeded and has been thinly sliced
- Two large eggs
- Four hundred grams of cherry tomatoes
- One small avocado that has been sliced
- One lime that has been cut into wedges

Method:

1. Heat the oil nicely in a big non-stick pan for some time.
2. Add the garlic and the chili to the heated oil and cook that for some time.
3. Take the two eggs and break them with caution on either side of the pan and let them set.

4. When the eggs start to set, take the beans and the cherry tomatoes and place them on the pan.

5. Sprinkle cumin seeds over all the ingredients in the pan.

6. Keep in mind that you want to warm the tomatoes and the beans and not cook them completely. So, keep them on the heat for as long as it is needed and not more than that.

7. When it is done, take the pan off the heat and then sprinkle the coriander and add the avocado over everything.

8. Squeeze the lemon wedges on top

9. Serve hot.

Note: Do not overcook the cherry tomatoes and the beans as that will take away the freshness from the dish.

3 pm – Chocolate Protein Shake

Total Time: 5 minutes

Yields: 1

Nutrition facts: Calories: 241 | Carbs: 28g | Protein: 26g | Fat: 3g | Fiber: 7g

Ingredients:

- Half cup of ice
- Three-fourth cup of almond milk
- Two tbsps. each of
    - Cocoa powder (unsweetened)
    - Hemp seeds (more may be required for serving)
    - Almond butter
- One tbsp. of chia seeds (more may be needed for serving)
- Half tbsp. of vanilla extract (pure)

- Two-three tbsps. of sugar substitute (keto-friendly)
- A pinch of kosher salt

Method:

1. Pour all the ingredients into a blender for combining appropriately. Keep blending until smooth.

2. After that, pour the protein shake into one large-sized glass.

3. Before serving, garnish with a little bit more hemp seeds and chia seeds. Enjoy!

5 pm – Caprese Chicken

Total Time: 40 minutes

Yields: 4

Nutrition Facts: Calories: 315 | Protein: 35.7g | Carbs: 1.63g | Fiber: 0.4g | Fat: 18.7g

Ingredients:

- Two tablespoons of avocado oil
- Salt and pepper according to taste
- One medium tomato that has been sliced in as many numbers as there are chicken thighs
- Five boneless chicken thighs with the removed skin
- Six ounces of fresh mozzarella cheese that have been sliced into five or six slices
- One-fourth cup of fresh basil.

Method:

1. Preheat the oven that you will be using to 375 degrees Fahrenheit.

2. In a big skillet and heat the oil over a medium to high flame till the oil starts shimmering.

3. Take the chicken thighs and sprinkle the salt and pepper on them. Then add it to the pan in a single layer.

4. Fry the chicken for about two to three minutes on each side till it turns golden brown, and then take the other side and do the same for another two to three minutes.

5. After that, take a medium-sized casserole and add the chicken on top of that in a single layer evenly.

6. On top of each chicken thigh piece, place a piece of mozzarella and a slice of tomato.

7. Bake this for half an hour until all the cheese has melted over the chicken and is now bubbling over it. Make sure the chicken is well cooked.

8. Turn on the broiler and then cook the chicken some more till the top portions become slightly brown in color.

9. Remove from the oven carefully and garnish with fresh basil leaves.

Note: *Do not hurry with the cooking time as otherwise the chicken will not be completely cooked from the inside.*

Day 3

11 am – Green Smoothie

Total Time: 10 minutes

Yields: 2

Nutrition Facts: Calories: 148 | Protein: 6g | Carbs: 10g | Fat: 10g | Fiber: 5g

Ingredients:

- A cup of sliced frozen strawberry
- Two cups of baby spinach
- Half cup of avocado chunks (frozen)
- One and a half cups of almond milk (unsweetened)
- Two tbsps. of hemp seeds
- Three drops of Lakanto Monkfruit extract

Method:

1. First, you need to take a clean blender and add all the ingredients required for preparing the green smoothie. You need to blend till it becomes smooth enough.

2. After that, take two glasses and divide the smoothie equally. Consume it immediately.

Note: You may avoid adding Lakanto Monkfruit extract to your smoothie if you do not wish to make it sweeter. Feel free to adjust the drops according to your preference for sweetness.

3 pm – Cheese Crisps

Total Time: 30 minutes

Yields: 12

Nutrition Facts: Calories: 31 | Protein: 2g | Carbs: 0g | Fiber: 0g | Fat: 2g

Ingredients:

- One teaspoon dried basil
- One cup of shredded parmesan cheese, which is about 100 grams

Method:

1. Preheat the oven to about 350 degrees Fahrenheit.
2. Line a baking sheet with parchment paper on it.
3. Take the parmesan cheese and pile it by the spoonful on the baking tray.
4. Take the backside of the spoon and flatten the cheese on the baking sheet evenly.
5. Sprinkle all the dried basil on the tray, and make sure you do that evenly.
6. You need to bake this for about five to seven minutes until the cheese has become golden brown and crispy on the edges.
7. Enjoy.

Note: Make sure you spread out the cheese evenly; otherwise, it will not be properly cooked.

5 pm – Arugula and Cauliflower Shrimp

Total time: 30 minutes

Yields: 4

Nutrition Facts: Calories:308 | Protien: 24g | Carbs: 13g | Fat: 18g | Fiber: 5g

Ingredients:

For the shrimp

- One tablespoon of paprika
- Half a teaspoon of cayenne pepper
- Freshly ground black pepper and salt
- One pound shrimp (peeled and deveined)
- Two teaspoons of garlic powder
- One tablespoon of extra-virgin olive oil

For the cauliflower grits

- Four cups of riced cauliflower
- Half a cup of goat cheese (crumbled)
- Freshly ground black pepper and salt
- One tablespoon of unsalted butter
- One cup of whole milk

For the garlic arugula

- Three very thinly sliced garlic cloves
- Freshly ground black pepper and salt as per taste
- One tablespoon of extra-virgin olive oil
- Four cups of baby arugula

Method:

For the spicy shrimp,

1. Take a large zip-top plastic bag and place the shrimp in that.

2. In a bowl take the garlic powder and the paprika and mix them nicely in it. Add the cayenne to it and mix it well.

3. Pour this mixture into the bag of shrimp and toss the bag really well. Toss the bag really well till all the shrimp are nicely covered with this paste.

4. Keep this bag of shrimp on the fridge for some time till you prepare the grits.

For the cauliflower grits,

1. Take a pot and over a medium heat melt the butter in it. Now add the cauliflower rice in it and cook for two minutes till it releases moisture.

2. Take half of the milk and stir it well, bringing it to shimmer. Simmer it for some time till the cauliflower absorbs some of the milk.

3. Now add the remaining milk and make it simmer till it becomes a thick creamy paste, for about ten minutes.

4. Add the cheese in it and add the salt and pepper to it.

For the garlic arugula,

1. Take a frying pan or a big skillet and heat olive oil in it. Over a medium heat, sautee the garlic in it for a minute.

2. After that, take the arugula and stir it in the olive oil for three minutes. Give salt and pepper as per taste.

3. Serve this by diving the grits among four plates and place a quarter of arugula on top and a quarter of shrimp.

Note: *The fresh the ingredients are, the tastier the dish will be. So, make sure to choose only the freshest of the ingredients you get.*

Day 4

11 am – Scrambled Eggs with Veggies and Toast

Total Time: 5 minutes

Yields: 2

Nutrition Facts: Calories: 194 | Carbs: 0.5g | Protein: 19g | Fat: 37g | Fiber: 0g

Ingredients –

- Three tablespoons of butter
- One small tomato that has been diced finely
- One-third cup of heavy cream
- Half a tablespoon of salt
- Two tablespoons of scallions that have been thinly sliced
- One serrano chili that has been finely chopped
- Four large eggs
- Two tablespoons of cilantro that has been finely chopped
- One pinch of pepper

Method:

1. Take a large non-stick frying pan and heat the butter over medium heat.
2. When the butter has been heated, add the chili and the tomato to it. Saute the chili and the tomato for about two minutes.
3. Take a mixing bowl, break the eggs and whisk them together with the cream, salt, and pepper according to taste and the cilantro.
4. Now pour the egg mixture into the frying pan and gently free the edges from the pan with the help of a flat spatula.

5. Then start drawing the eggs towards the center and then allow the eggs to get settled around the edges.

6. Repeat the same process till the eggs become a soft scramble.

7. Cook the eggs for some time over the heat till they are not runny anymore and they become a soft scramble.

8. Add the scallions and serve hot.

Note: *Make sure the eggs are as fresh as possible to take the best and the soft scrambled eggs.*

3 pm – Yogurt Granola Parfait

Total Time: 5 minutes

Yields: 1

Nutrition Facts: Calories: 436 | Protein: 8.2g | Carbs: 19.6g | Fat: 38.1g | Fiber: 7.9g

Ingredients:

- Half a cup of coconut yogurt
- Eight raspberries
- One-fourth cup of fresh blueberries
- One teaspoon of hemp hearts
- One-fourth cup of vanilla maple keto granola
- Two strawberries cut in half
- One teaspoon of chia seeds
- Fresh mint for garnishing

Method:

1. Take a bowl big enough to fit all the ingredients.

2. Add the coconut yogurt and all the other ingredients one after the other.

3. Put the fresh mint on top for garnishing.

Note: This recipe is all about what you like to add, so make sure to add things that you prefer to have in the mornings to give your day a fresh start.

5 pm – Smoked Salmon and Avocado

Total Time: 5 minutes

Yields: 2

Nutrition Facts: Calories: 548 | Proteins: 25g | Carbs: 4g | Fat: 45g | Fiber: 1g

Ingredients:

- Eight ounces of smoked salmon
- Two avocadoes, that is, fourteen ounces of avocadoes
- Salt and pepper according to taste
- Two tablespoons of mayonnaise

Method:

1. At first, take the avocadoes and split them in half. Remove the pit from inside it and then scoop out the entire avocado with the help of a spoon.
2. Place the avocadoes on a plate and keep them aside.
3. Now, take the salmon and the mayonnaise and add them to the plate.
4. Finally, add salt and pepper according to taste on top of it.

Note: Try to get as fresh salmon as possible as that changes the taste completely and uplifts the dish.

Day 5

11 am – Blackberry Chia Pudding

Total Time: 30 minutes

Yields: 4

Nutrition Facts: Calories: 201 | Carbs: 4.2g | Protein: 5.2g | Fat: 14.9g | Fiber: 9.6g

Ingredients:

- Half a cup of chia seeds
- Two tablespoons of MCT oil or walnut oil, or macadamia oil
- One teaspoon of sugar-free vanilla extract
- One teaspoon of ground cinnamon
- One tablespoon of powdered erythritol or swerve or stevia drops
- Two and a half cups of unsweetened almond milk
- One cup of fresh blackberries or even frozen and thawed blackberries will do
- One and a half teaspoons of ground cardamom
- Half teaspoon of ground ginger
- Coconut cream (optional)

Method:

1. Take all the ingredients but the chia seeds in a blender and blend them well.
2. Make sure the mixture is completely smooth, and then pour this mixture on top of the chia seeds.
3. Give this a good stir, and let this soak well for at least half an hour.
4. Make sure the bowl is well covered while it is resting.

5. You can also put this in your fridge overnight.

6. When you want to serve it, add the almond milk to make it of your desired consistency.

Note: You can store this for up to five days in your fridge.

3 pm – Zuppa Toscana Soup

Total Time: 30 minutes

Yields: 6

Nutrition Facts: Calories: 260m| Protein: 19g | Carbs: 9g | Fat: 18g | Fiber: 2g

Ingredients:

- Four slices of bacon
- One large onion, finely diced
- Six cups of low sodium chicken broth
- Two cups of chopped kale, either fresh or frozen
- Half a teaspoon of black pepper
- Freshly grated parmesan for serving
- Three cloves of garlic that has been minced
- 1 lb of ground turkey sausage
- One head cauliflower finely chopped
- Three fourth cup of heavy cream
- Kosher salt according to taste

Method:

1. Take a large pot or a dutch oven and heat it over medium flame for some time.

2. Saute the bacon slices over it until they are crispy.

3. Take out the bacon and set them aside for some time. Leave the bacon fat on the pan itself.

4. In that heated pan with the bacon fat, add the garlic and the onion and fry them till they are completely translucent for about five minutes.

5. Now add the sausages to the pan and take a spatula to break them apart to get a nice crumble. Cook it thoroughly for about five minutes.

6. When it has been cooked properly, add the chicken broth, kale, pepper, and cauliflower to it. Let this get cooked properly for about ten minutes. Make sure the cauliflower is well cooked and can be broken with a fork easily.

7. Now that everything is cooked stir the entire thing after adding the heavy cream to it and add the seasonings to it.

8. Add salt according to taste.

9. While serving, add the bacon and the parmesan cheese to it.

Note: In order to make the preparation of the meal easier, use frozen chopped kale, already minced garlic, and frozen diced onion.

5 pm – Greek Salmon Bowl

Total Time: 45 minutes

Yields: 4

Nutrition Facts: Calories: 484 | Carbs: 28g | Protein: 30g | Fat: 28g | Fiber: 4g

Ingredients:

- One pound salmon fillet
- One-fourth teaspoon of ground pepper
- One and a third cups of water
- Three tablespoons of lemon juice

- Two teaspoons of finely crushed oregano for the cooking and half a teaspoon of crushed oregano for garnishing
- One-fourth cup of crumbled feta cheese
- Half a teaspoon of salt
- Eight ounces of string beans that can be green or yellow or even mixed. Trim them into one-inch pieces
- Three-fourth cup of quinoa (can be red or white, or tricolored) Rinse them properly
- Two tablespoons of olive oil
- One clove of garlic that has been minced
- One medium-sized tomato that has been seeded and chopped
- One-fourth cup of pitted kalamata olives that have been halved or sliced

Method:

1. Preheat the oven to 400 degrees Fahrenheit. Take a large baking sheet and line it with foil.
2. Place a salmon on this baking tray and sprinkle about one-eighth of a teaspoon of salt on it.
3. Bake the salmon until the fish is no longer opaque in the center region and it starts to flakes easily.
4. Bake the fish for about half an hour and then let it rest for about five minutes, and then use a fork to flake the fish into small bite-size pieces.
5. Take another saucepan to boil about one inch of water in it. Make sure a steamer basket is fitted with this saucepan.
6. Add the beans and then cover the pan and cook the beans until they are tender and crisp. Cook this for about five minutes.
7. Wash these beans under cold water and drain the water well, and then set the beans aside.

8. Take the quinoa and one-eight teaspoon of salt in the saucepan and boil it. Reduce the heat, and then let the quinoa simmer for some time until it is tender and almost all the liquid has been absorbed. Keep this on the heat for about 15 to 20 minutes, and then fluff it with a fork.

9. Take the lemon juice and whisk it well with the garlic, oregano, oil, and the remaining amount of salt.

10. While serving, divide the quinoa into four bowls and arrange everything, that is, the salmon, tomatoes, feta, beans, and olives over the quinoa.

Note: *While serving, make sure to drizzle some more fresh oregano over the top for better taste.*

Day 6

11 am – Low Carb Muesli

Total Time: 9 minutes

Yields: 15

Nutrition Facts: Calories: 217 | Carbs: 6g | Protein: 8g | Fat: 19g | Fiber: 3g

Ingredients:

- One cup each of
    - Sliced almonds
    - Pumpkin seeds
    - Flaked coconut (unsweetened)
    - Sunflower seeds
- Two tsps. of cinnamon
- Half cup each of
    - Hemp hearts
    - Pecans
- A quarter tsp. of stevia drops (vanilla)
- Half tsp. of vanilla extract

Method:

1. First of all, you need to take one large-sized bowl. Pour every single ingredient into the bowl and stir by using a spatula. Stirring helps combine all the ingredients properly.

2. Next, you need to take one baking pan (rimmed) and place the mixed ingredients in it. In the meantime, set the temperature of your oven to 350 degrees. Insert the pan and bake for nearly eight minutes.

3. Once the baking is done, let it cool. You may store it in any container (air-tight).

4. One serving is almost one-third cup, and the taste enhances if almond milk is added to it.

3 pm – Rosemary Crackers

Total Time: 1 hour

Yields: 140

Nutrition Facts: Calories: 27 | Carbs: 4g | Protein: 0.7g | Fat: 0.8g | Fiber: 0.2g

Ingredients:

- Half cup of coconut flour
- Two and a half cups of almond flour
- Half tsp. each of
    - Onion powder
    - Chopped dried rosemary
- One tsp. of flaxseed meal (ground)
- Three large-sized eggs
- One tbsp. of olive oil (Extra-virgin)
- A quarter tsp. of kosher salt

Method:

1. At first, the oven needs to be preheated by setting the temperature to 325 degrees. Meanwhile, take parchment paper for lining one baking sheet. Whisk flax meal, coconut flour, almond flour, onion powder, rosemary, and salt together in one large bowl. Then, add in oil and eggs and combine all the ingredients evenly. You have to mix it continuously till the dough takes the shape of one large ball.

2. Now, you have to sandwich the dough that you have made in between two parchment pieces of paper and then roll to a thickness of one-fourth inch. After that, use a knife for cutting into squares. Transfer all the squares to the baking sheet that you have prepared in the beginning.

3. Bake for almost fifteen minutes till the crackers attain a golden color. You can store the crackers in any resealable container, but before that, it is necessary to cool them properly.

5 pm – Fish Taco Bowl

Total Time: 21 minutes

Yields: 4

Nutrition Facts: Calories: 370 | Protein: 36g | Carbs: 13g | Fat: 21g | Fiber: 6g

Ingredients:

- One and a half pounds of halibut or cod fillets.
- Two tablespoons of taco seasoning
- One yellow bell pepper that has been julienned
- One avocado that has been peeled, pitted, and also sliced
- One cup of nicely shredded red cabbage
- Ground black pepper and sea salt according to taste
- Lime wedges for garnishing
- One-fourth cup of finely sliced black olives
- Fresh cilantro for garnishing
- One cup of cherry tomatoes cut in halves
- One jalapeno pepper that has been sliced
- Two cups of lime cauliflower rice and cilantro

- Three tablespoons of olive oil

Method:

1. In the beginning, cut the fish into four almost equal-sized pieces and place the pieces on a shallow baking dish.

2. Add a generous amount of olive oil and taco seasonings to the pieces making sure they are well quoted.

3. Set them aside for some time while you prepare the rest of the dish.

4. Take the four serving bowls and place half a cup of cauliflower rice in each of them.

5. Then, arrange one quarter each of jalapeno, tomatoes, olives, bell pepper, avocado, cabbage around the outside of the bowl while making sure to leave a place in the middle.

6. Take a grilling pan and heat it over medium heat for some time. After the pan is hot, place the fish on the pan and cook for some time until it becomes brown and flakes easily.

7. Cook the fish for about three minutes on each side.

8. Now when the fish is done, place one piece each in that space that you had earlier created while arranging the bowls.

9. Garnish the bowls with cilantro and when you serve it, add the lime wedges.

Note: You can store all the leftovers in your fridge for about three days. Instead of cauliflower rice, you can also use steamed white rice if you want to reduce the calory further. Some might not be fish eaters, and in that case, feel free to use chicken or beef in place of fish.

Day 7

11 am – Hemp Seed Oatmeal

Total Time: 10 minutes

Yields: 2

Nutrition Facts: Calories: 432 | Carbs: 15.2g | Protein: 11.6g | Fat: 39g | Fiber: 10.7g

Ingredients:

- One tbsp. of flaxseed
- A quarter cup each of
    - Chia seeds
    - Hemp Heart seeds
- One cup of coconut milk or almond milk
- Two tbsps. of erythritol

Method:

1. Take a small-sized saucepan and place every single ingredient into it. Keep the saucepan on top of your oven and set medium heat. You need to keep stirring till you get to see a properly blended mixture.

2. Heat it gently for approximately three to five minutes.

3. After you are done with this part, if you notice that the mixture has turned out to be very stiff, simply add almond milk and that too in a very small quantity.

4. You may serve this dish immediately.

3 pm – Bacon Guac Bombs

Total Time: 45 minutes

Yields: 15

Nutrition Facts: Calories: 156 | Carbs: 1.4g | Protein: 3.4g | Fat: 15.2g | Fiber: 1.3g

Ingredients:

- Twelve bacon slices (crumbled and cooked)

For preparing Guacamole

- Six ounces of softened cream cheese
- Two avocados (peeled, pitted, and mashed)
- One clove of garlic (minced)
- One lime juice
- One small-sized jalapeno (chopped)
- A quarter minced red onion
- Half tsp. each of
    - Chili powder
    - Cumin
- Two tbsps. of cilantro (freshly chopped)
- Black pepper (freshly ground)
- Kosher salt

Method:

1. At first, you need to take one large-sized mixing bowl to combine all the ingredients of guacamole. Keep stirring till the mixture becomes smooth (a few chunks won't cause any problem), and then season with pepper and salt. Transfer the bowl to the refrigerator and keep it inside for half an hour.

2. Now, take one large plate and keep the crumbled bacon on it. Use one small-sized cookie scoop for scooping the already prepared guacamole mixture. Place one scoop of mixture in each bacon and then roll for coating in bacon. Repeat the same process till all the bacon, and the entire quantity of guacamole mixture are used up. Store in your refrigerator.

5 pm - Wild Cajun Spicy Salmon

Total Time: 30 minutes

Yields: 4

Nutrition Facts: Calories: 408 | Carbs: 9g | Protein: 42g | Fat: 23g | Fiber: 3g

Ingredients:

- Half lb. of head cauliflower (chopped into florets)
- One and a half lb. of salmon fillets (wild Alaskan)
- One lb. of head broccoli (chopped into florets)
- Four medium-sized diced tomatoes
- Half tsp. of garlic powder
- Three tbsps. of olive oil
- Taco seasoning (sodium-free)

Method:

1. At first, the oven needs to be preheated and for that, set the temperature of your oven to exactly 375 degrees. Keep the fillets of salmon in one baking dish. Next, you need to take one small-sized bowl and combine half a cup of water and taco seasoning in it. Once the mixing is done, pour it over the fillets and let it bake for nearly fifteen minutes or till the salmon becomes opaque throughout.

2. In the meantime, pulse both broccoli and cauliflower by using a food processor until the veggies become evenly chopped as well as riced.

3. Now, take one large-sized skillet and heat olive oil over medium heat. When the oil becomes hot, add in the chopped broccoli and cauliflower and then sprinkle garlic powder. Toss and cook until all the ingredients become tender or for about five to six minutes.

4. Lastly, place the baked salmon fillets on top of the rice. Top with the diced tomatoes and serve.

Day 8

11 am – Easy Shakshuka

Total Time: 50 minutes

Yields: 4

Nutrition Facts: Calories: 157 | Protein: 10g | Carbs: 11.9g | Fat: 6.9g | Fiber: 3.7g

Ingredients:

- Two chopped garlic cloves
- One red chili that has been deseeded and chopped finely
- One green pepper finely chopped
- One teaspoon of ground turmeric
- Two tins of tomatoes of 400g each, finely chopped
- Handful of coriander
- Two teaspoons of Nigella seed
- One chopped onion
- A thumb-sized piece of well-chopped ginger
- Two teaspoons of vegetable oil

- Two teaspoons of ground turmeric
- One teaspoon of ground coriander
- A handful of baby spinach
- Four small eggs

Method:

1. Take a blender and put the onions, chili, garlic and tomatoes, and ginger and blend them into a nice and smooth paste.

2. Take a frying pan of about 30cm deep and heat oil in it.

3. Add the puree that you just made in it and fry it well for some time.

4. Add green pepper to it and the seasonings as well.

5. Cook it till the raw smell of the vegetables doesn't come anymore.

6. Take the cumin, ground coriander, and turmeric and stir them well and then add the tinned tomatoes to it.

7. Add 100 ml of water to it and let it simmer for about twenty minutes.

8. Stir the spinach and the chopped coriander and cook for some time.

9. When it is cooked well, make four pockets in the pan and gently break the eggs in those pockets.

10. Put the lid on and let the eggs get cooked for some time.

11. It will take about ten to eleven minutes for the entire dish to get cooked completely.

12. When you serve the dish, sprinkle the nigella seeds on top.

3 pm – Avocado Chips

Total Time: 40 minutes

Yields: 15

Nutrition facts: Calories: 120 | Carbs: 4g | Protein: 7g | Fat: 10g | Fiber: 2g

Ingredients:

- Three-forth cup of Parmesan (freshly grated)
- One large-sized ripe avocado
- Half tsp. each of
    - Italian seasoning
    - Garlic powder
- One tsp. of lemon juice
- Black pepper (freshly ground)
- Kosher salt

Method:

1. In the beginning, preheat your oven by setting the temperature to 325 degrees. Take two baking sheets and use parchment paper for lining both of them. Now, take one medium-sized bowl and a fork for mashing avocado until smooth. As you are done with the mashing part, stir in lemon juice, Parmesan, Italian seasoning, and garlic powder. You need to do the seasoning with pepper and salt.

2. Scoop teaspoon size heaps of the prepared mixture on the lined baking sheet. You need to make sure that there is a gap of three inches between each scoop. Next, take a measuring cup or spoon and use its backside for flattening each scoop having a width of three inches. Place the baking sheet inside the oven and allow it to bake for half an hour until golden and crisp. Take out the

sheet from the oven and let it cool completely. Satisfy your taste buds by serving at usual room temperature.

5 pm – Fried Chicken with Broccoli

Total Time: 20 minutes

Yields: 2

Nutrition Facts: Calories: 484 | Protein: 43g | Carbs: 5g | Fat: 31g | Fiber: 2g

Ingredients:

- Two ounces of butter
- Salt and pepper according to taste
- Nine ounces of broccoli
- Fourteen ounces of chicken thighs (boneless)

Method:

1. Take the broccoli and wash it properly. After you have rinsed them well, trim them.
2. Keep in mind to keep the stems intact and cut them into small pieces.
3. Take a frying pan and heat up the butter in it. Keep in mind that the butter should be enough to fry both the broccoli and the chicken in it.
4. Season the chicken from beforehand.
5. Now take the chicken and fry it in the butter. Fry each side for five minutes over medium heat.
6. Fry the chicken until it is golden brown in color. Make sure it is cooked completely.
7. After the chicken has been fried properly, add some butter and then add the broccoli to the pan.
8. Fry for some more minutes.

9. Pepper and salt should be added as per your taste.

10. Serve when hot and enjoy!

Note: You can also make this dish with many other vegetables which have a low carbohydrate content, like zucchini or spinach, or asparagus. It completely depends on you as to which vegetable you will use. Also, feel free to add your favorite spices for more flavor, like onion powder. You could also add different herbs and paprika if you want.

Day 9

11 am – Egg Wraps with Greens and Ham

Total time: 20 minutes

Yield: 4

Nutritional Facts: Calories: 371 | Carbs: 4.9g| Fat: 26.5g | Fiber: 0.5g | Protein: 27.4g

Ingredients:

- Eight eggs
- Two teaspoons of all-purpose flour or cornstarch
- Four teaspoons of water
- Four teaspoons of vegetable oil or even coconut oil will work
- ½ teaspoon of fine salt
- 1 1/3 cups of swiss cheese (shred them)
- 1 1/3 cups of watercress (loosely packed)
- 4 ounces of ham (slice them thinly)

Method:

1. Take a medium bowl and add eggs, flour or cornstarch, water, and salt in it and whisk it until the flor or the cornstarch is totally dissolved.

2. Add one teaspoon of oil to a 12-inch nonstick frying pan and heat the oil heat over medium flame. Swirl the oil to make sure that the bottom of the pan is covered with oil. Now add ½ cups of egg mixture into the frying pan and swirl to coat the bottom of the pan so that it forms a thin layer. Cook for 3 to 6 minutes till the egg is completely set on the edges.

3. Use a flat spatula and try to loosen the sides of the wrap, and make sure that you can flip it easily. After flipping it, add cheese on top of it and cook for about 1 minute. Now transfer it to a cutting board and put ham on top of it, also at 1/3 cup of watercress at the center of the wrap and roll it tightly.

4. Repeat the same process with the rest of the wraps. Cut each wrap to 6 pieces with a knife and serve hot.

3 pm – Ice Cream

Total Time: 8 hours 15 minutes

Yields: 8

Nutrition Facts: Calories: 279 | Carbs: 36g | Protein: 3.3g | Fat: 15g | Fiber: 2g

Ingredients:

-   Two cups of heavy cream
-   Two 15-ounce cans of coconut milk
-   One tsp. of vanilla extract (pure)
-   A quarter cup of sweetener
-   A pinch of Kosher salt

Method:

1. Before you start preparing this mouth-watering ice cream, you have to keep the coconut milk inside the refrigerator for a minimum time of three hours or, ideally, overnight.

2. For making whipped coconut, you need to take one large-sized bowl and spoon out coconut cream in it and leave the liquid inside the can. After that, take one hand mixer and use it for beating coconut cream till it becomes very creamy. Keep it aside.

3. The next step is to prepare the whipped cream. For that, take one separate large-sized bowl and hand mixer. Beat the heavy cream in it till you get to see the formation of very soft peaks. Then, beat in vanilla and sweetener.

4. Your next step is to fold the already prepared whipped coconut into the whipped cream. Now, transfer the entire mixture into one loaf pan.

5. Put the pan in your refrigerator and let it freeze for almost five hours until solid.

5 pm – Turkey Tacos

Total Time: 25 minutes

Yields: 4

Nutrition Facts: Calories: 472 | Carbs: 30g | Protein: 28g | Fat: 27g | Fiber: 6g

Ingredients:

- One lb. of ground turkey (extra-lean)
- One small-sized chopped red onion
- Two tsps. of oil
- One finely chopped clove of garlic
- One sliced avocado
- Eight corn tortillas (whole-grain, warmed)
- One tbsp. of taco seasoning (sodium-free)
- A quarter cup of sour cream

- One cup of chopped lettuce

- Half cup of Mexican cheese (shredded)

- Salsa (required for serving)

Method:

1. First of all, you need to take one large-sized skillet and pour oil into it. Heat the poured oil over medium to high flame. Next, you have to add the chopped onion and stir for about five to six minutes until tender. Once the onion becomes tender, add in the chopped garlic. Stir and cook for a minute.

2. Now, you need to add one lb. of turkey and use a spoon to break it evenly. Cook for almost five minutes until the turkey becomes nearly brown. Then, you have to add a cup of water and taco seasoning. Let it simmer for about six to seven minutes until it gets decreased to almost half portion.

3. Next, it is time to fill in the tortillas with cooked turkey. Top with cheese, salsa, avocado, sour cream, and lettuce.

Day 10

11 am – Avocado Toasts with Poached Eggs

Total Time: 15 minutes

Yields: 4

Nutrition Facts: Calories: 439.8 | Carbs: 26.6g | Protein: 16.2g | Fat: 31.2g | Fiber: 7.5g

Ingredients:

- Two ripe avocados
- Four thick slices of bread
- Two tsps. of lemon juice/ juice of one lime
- Four eggs
- One cup of cheese (grated, gruyere, edam, or any other present on hand)
- Four tsps. of butter (to spread on toast)
- Black pepper (freshly ground)
- Salt (as required)

Method:

1. At first, you need to poach the eggs with the help of your favorite process.
2. In the meantime, slice the ripe avocados in equal halves, as well as take out the stones.
3. After that, take a clean spoon of large size for scooping out its flesh. As you are done with the scooping part, keep the flesh of the avocado into one bowl. Now, it is time to add the lime or lemon juice as well as the required quantity of ground black pepper and salt.
4. The next step is to use a fork for mashing all the ingredients roughly that are inside the bowl.

5. Once you finish mashing, toast the slices of bread—spread butter on top of each slice.

6. Now, you need to take a sufficient amount of avocado mix to spread it onto every single buttered toast slice. Top each slice with one poached egg.

7. For additional taste, sprinkle grated cheese over the poached eggs. Serve it immediately.

Note: For enhancing the taste, you may include either grilled or fresh tomato halves beside the avocado toasts.

3 pm – Carrot Cake

Total time: 55 minutes

Yield: 16

Nutritional Facts: Calories: 359 | Protein: 7.5g | Fat: 34g | Carbs: 8.5g | Fiber: 3g

Ingredients:

- ¾ cup of best erythritol or coconut sugar
- One tablespoon of Blackstrap molasses
- Four eggs
- ¾ cup of butter
- One teaspoon of vanilla extract
- ½ teaspoon of pineapple extract
- 2 ½ cups of almond flour
- Two teaspoons of cinnamon
- Two teaspoons of baking powder
- 2 ½ cups of grated carrot
- 1 ½ cups of chopped pecans

- ½ teaspoon of sea salt
- Two cream cheese frosting (sugar-free)

Method:

1. Prepare two in 9 in round cake pans with parchment paper. Grease the bottom and the side. Also, preheat the oven to 350 degrees Fahrenheit before cooking.

2. Take a large bowl and mix the butter and the erythritol until the cream becomes fluffy. Also, beat the eggs, one at a time, and the molasses, pineapple extracts, and vanilla extract.

3. Take another bowl and add almond flour, cinnamon, baking powder, and sea salt and mix them. Now stir the dry and wet ingredients together in one bowl.

4. Stir the carrots and fold 1 cup of pecans which you have grated beforehand.

5. Take two baking pans and transfer the batter to it. Now bake for 30 to 35 mins.

6. Cool the cakes for 10 minutes.

7. When the cake has cooled down, transfer it to a plate, slice it and top it with chopped pecans.

5 pm – Fried Cauliflower Rice with Chicken

Total time: 35 minutes

Yields: 4

Nutrition Facts: Calories: 427 | Carbs: 25g | Protein: 45g | Fat: 16g | Fiber: 7g

Ingredients:

- Four large-sized eggs (beaten)
- One and a half lb. of skinless, boneless chicken breast (crushed to uniform thickness)

- Two small-sized carrots (chopped finely)
- Two bell peppers (red, finely chopped)
- Two finely chopped cloves of garlic
- One onion (chopped finely)
- Half cup of thawed, frozen peas
- Four cups of cauliflower rice
- Four finely chopped scallions
- Two tbsps. each of
  - Soy sauce (low-sodium)
  - Grapeseed oil
- Two tsps. of rice vinegar
- Pepper and Kosher salt

Method:

1. Take one deep and large-sized skillet and set the heat to medium temperature. Pour one tbsp. of oil and heat it. Once the oil becomes hot enough, add the entire quantity of chicken. Cook each side for three to four minutes till the color turns golden brown. Now, you need to transfer the cooked or fried chicken to your cutting board. Before you start slicing the chicken, allow it to rest for about five to six minutes. Pour one tbsp. of oil into the skillet and add the beaten eggs for scrambling. You might need one to two minutes to cook the scrambled eggs. Transfer it to a small-sized bowl.

2. Now, you need to add carrot, onion, and bell pepper to the same skillet and cook for nearly four to five minutes. You need to stir all the ingredients quite often till all of them become tender. As soon as you get to see the tender texture, stir in the finely chopped garlic cloves and cook for one more minute. It is time to toss with thawed peas and scallions.

3. After that, add soy sauce, rice vinegar, cauliflower, pepper, and salt, and tossing is required for combining all the ingredients properly. Do not stir for two to three minutes so that the cauliflower begins to get the brown color and also gets the time to sit. Lastly, you need to toss with scrambled eggs and sliced chicken.

Day 11

11 am – Almond Vanilla Granola

Total Time: 2 hours 10 minutes

Yields: 12

Nutrition Facts: Calories: 187.1 | Carbs: 25.3g | Protein: 3.9g | Fat: 8g | Fiber: 2.9g

Ingredients:

- Half cup each of
    - Cane sugar (natural)
    - Water
    - Sliced almonds
- Three and a half cups of oats (old fashioned)
- A quarter cup of grapeseed oil or a quarter cup of canola oil (organic)
- A quarter tsp. of salt
- One tbsp. of vanilla extract

Method:

1. For heating, your oven set the temperature to exactly 200 degrees. Use parchment paper for lining one rimmed cookie sheet of large size.

2. Now, take one large bowl and place the almonds and oats into it. Mix both the ingredients together.

3. Pour salt and cane sugar along with water into one small saucepan and put it over almost medium heat. Keep stirring. The stirring should be continued till the sugar gets dissolved completely. Remove the saucepan from heat. Next, pour in and stir vanilla and canola oil. You also need to pour the almond and oats mixture into the same saucepan. You need to check whether all the ingredients have been thoroughly combined or not; stirring is necessary till then.

4. After that, spread the combined mixture properly on the already lined cookie sheet. Put it inside the preheated oven and bake it for almost two hours. Or, the baking needs to be done until it is super dry for touching. You must not stir at all in this stage. Then the sheet needs to be removed from the oven. Allow it to cool completely, and only then will you be able to break it into chunks. Lastly, store the chunks in a container (air-tight).

3 pm – Chocolate Mousse

Total Time: 10 minutes

Yields: 4

Nutrition facts: Calories: 218 | Carbs: 5g | Protein: 2g | Fat: 23g | Fiber: 2g

Ingredients:

- A quarter cup each of
  - Powdered sweetener
  - Cocoa powder (unsweetened, sifted)
- One cup of whipping cream (heavy)
- One tsp. of vanilla extract
- A quarter tsp. of kosher salt

Method:

1. The very first step of making chocolate mousse is whisking the entire quantity of cream till it becomes thick. For whisking, you may opt for either any hand mixer or stand mixer.

2. Next, you have to add sweetener, cocoa powder, salt, and vanilla extract. Keep whisking till the ingredients are combined smoothly.

Note: Those who are willing to make a bit lighter mousse must whisk the egg whites of three large-sized eggs to firm peaks. Then, it must be folded into your mousse mixture for combining as required.

5 pm – Turkey Meatballs with Zucchini Pasta

Turkey Meatballs

Total time: Turkey meatballs: 40 minutes

Yield: 20

Nutritional Facts: Calories: 134 | Carbs: 1g | Protein: 12g | Fat: 10g | Fiber: 1g

Ingredients:

- 2 lbs of ground turkey
- ¼ cup of nutritional yeast
- One egg
- ½ sliced bell pepper
- 1 cup of finely chopped spinach
- One teaspoon of garlic powder or one tablespoon of garlic oil
- ¼ cup of freshly chopped parsley
- ½ teaspoon of ground black pepper

- ½ teaspoon of sea salt

For the spice aioli sauce

- One egg
- ¾ cup of avocado oil
- One tablespoon of hot sauce
- ½ teaspoon of mustard powder
- ¼ teaspoon of sea salt

Method:

1. Line a large baking sheet with parchment paper and preheat the oven to 400 degrees Fahrenheit.

2. Use your hand to mix and combine all the ingredients in a big mixing bowl.

3. Mix them well and form into meatballs in the size of an oversized golf ball and place them on a lined baking sheet.

4. Transfer the meatballs into the oven and bake it for 20 to 25 minutes until it is cooked completely. You could also switch the oven to broil for about 2 to 3 minutes, in the end, to make the top of the meatballs look brown.

5. While the meatballs are baking, prepare the sauce. Choose a container big enough to immerse your blender. Put all the ingredients for the sauce in the container.

6. Now put the blender in the container and start blending everything. Make sure that the sauce gets thick and begins to emulsify. Make sure that the oil is also totally mixed. The sauce should be creamy and store in the refrigerator until you use it.

7. Once your meatballs are cooked, remove them from the oven and serve them with spicy aioli sauce.

Note: *Making the sauce is totally optional; you can choose not to make it, but the meatballs taste great with the aioli sauce.*

Zucchini Pasta

Total time*:* 15 minutes

Yield: 1

Nutritional value: Calories: 157 | Fat: 13.9g | Protein: 2.9g | Carbs: 7.9g | Fiber: 2g

Ingredients:

- 2 peeled zucchinis
- ¼ cup of water
- One tablespoon of olive oil
- Salt
- Ground black pepper

Method:

1. Cut the zucchini, slice them lengthwise, using a vegetable peeler, and stop when the seeds are reached. Slice the zucchini into thinner strips so that it resembles spaghetti

2. Heat olive oil in a pan over medium heat and stir the zucchini in the hot oil for 1 minute.

3. Add water to it and cook until it becomes soft (for about 5 to 7 minutes)

4. Season with salt and pepper. Your zucchini pasta is ready

Note: You could also make a sauce with it, but since you are going to eat it with the turkey meatballs, you probably will not need it.

Day 12

11 am – Peach Berry Smoothie

Total Time: 5 minutes

Yields: 1

Nutrition Facts: Calories: 351.3 | Carbs: 61.6g | Protein: 2.7g | Fat: 12.4g | Fiber: 4.5g

Ingredients:

- One cup full of frozen peaches
- Half cup of Greek yogurt
- A quarter cup of coconut milk
- Half tsp. of almond flavoring

Method:

1. Take one blender of high speed and pour the entire quantity of frozen peaches and almond flavoring into it. Let it blend or mix well.

2. After that, you need to check the thickness of the smoothie so that you can adjust it accordingly. If you want your peach berry smoothie to be thinner, then you need to add in more milk. But, if your preference is to enjoy a thicker one, you better add more peaches. Pour it into a medium-sized bowl.

3. Before serving, top it with attractive and tasty toppings such as berries, slivered almonds, and chia seeds.

4. Lastly, enjoy the creamy, sweet bowl of smoothies so that your day starts in the perfect healthy manner.

3 pm – Pistachio Avocado Toast

Total time: 15 minutes

Yield: 1

Nutritional Facts: Calories: 376 | Carbs: 11g | Fat: 38g | Protein: 5g | Fiber: 8g

Ingredients:

- One slice of keto bread
- ½ tablespoon of lime juice
- ½ of ripe avocado
- 1/8 tomato (dice them)
- Two tablespoons of olive oil
- Six crushed pistachios
- Sea salt

Method:

1. Toast one slice of keto bread properly.
2. Cut the avocado into two halves and drizzle lime juice on top of it.
3. Now smash the avocado on top of the toasted bread and spread it evenly.
4. Sprinkle the crushed pistachios, chopped tomatoes, and sea salt on top of the avocados.
5. Drizzle the olive oil over the avocado toast.
6. Enjoy your toast with a fork and knife, or eat it by using your hands.

Note: The olive oil that you are using could be extra virgin olive oil as that will make the dish even healthier.

5 pm – Spaghetti Bolognese

Total Time: One and a half hours

Yields: 4

Nutrition Facts: Calories: 450 | Carbs: 31g | Protein: 32g | Fat: 23g | Fiber: 6g

Ingredients:

- One and a quarter lb. of ground turkey
- One large-sized spaghetti squash
- Half tsp. of garlic powder
- Three tbsps. of olive oil
- One small-sized finely chopped onion
- Four finely chopped garlic cloves
- Three cups or two 15-ounce cans of diced tomatoes (fresh)
- Eight ounces of small-sized and sliced cremini mushrooms
- Basil (freshly chopped)
- One 8 ounce can of tomato sauce (sugarless and low-sodium)
- Pepper and Kosher salt

Method:

1. First of all, you need to preheat your oven by setting the temperature to exactly 400 degrees. Meanwhile, halve the large-sized spaghetti squash lengthwise and also discard the seeds. After that, rub every single half with half tbsp. of oil as well as season the halves with a quarter tsp. each of pepper and salt along with garlic powder. Take a baking sheet (rimmed) and place the seasoned spaghetti squash on it with the skin side upwards. Let it roast for more than half an hour, say about forty minutes or until tender. Once the roasting is done, allow cooling for the next ten minutes.

2. In the meantime, take one skillet of large size and heat two tbsps. of oil over medium heat. As soon as the oil becomes hot, add the finely chopped onion in it after seasoning with a quarter tsp. each of pepper and salt. Stir occasionally and cook for about six minutes until the onions become tender. Next, you need to add in the turkey and use a spoon to break it into very small pieces. Cook until it turns brown, or for seven minutes. After this, you also need to add in chopped garlic cloves and stir for a minute.

3. Now, you have to set aside the already prepared turkey mixture to a side and place the cremini mushrooms on the other side of the pan. Stir occasionally and cook for almost five minutes so that the mushrooms become perfectly tender. Now, mix it with the turkey and add tomato sauce and tomatoes into it. Let it simmer for approximately ten minutes.

4. When you observe the sauce simmering, you have to transfer the squash to plates after scooping it out. Pour the Turkey Bolognese on top. If you feel like it, you may sprinkle basil before serving.

Day 13

11 am – Capicola Egg Cups

Total time: 20 mins

Yield: 6

Nutritional Facts: Calories: 302 | Carbs: 3g | Protein: 24g | Fat: 21g | Fiber: 1g

Ingredients:

- 3 oz. of bacon and capicola (slice them)
- ¾ cups or 3 oz. of shredded cheddar cheese
- Six eggs
- If you want to garnish, then you need thinly chopped basil
- Salt
- Pepper

Method:

1. You need nonstick cooking spray and have to spray that to 6 wells of a standard-sized muffin pan.
2. Preheat the oven to 200 degrees Celcius or 400 degrees Fahrenheit.
3. Now you have to place the capicola in the six greased wells. Also, if you are using cheese, then you could spread two tablespoons of cheese in each and every cup.
4. Season the eggs with salt and pepper and fill the cups.
5. In the last step, you have to bake it until the egg whites are set. It will take approximately 12 to 14 minutes to bake properly. Garnish it with sliced basil and serve hot.

Note: You could use a muffin pan, and that would make the cooking process easier.

3 pm – Brown Butter Pralines

Total Time: 16 minutes

Yields: 10

Nutrition facts: Calories: 338 | Carbs: 3g | Protein: 2g | Fat: 36g | Fiber: 2g

Ingredients:

- Two cups of chopped pecans
- Two sticks of salted butter
- Two-third cups each of
  - Granular sweetener
  - Heavy cream
- Half tsp. of xanthan gum
- Sea salt (as required)

Method:

1. At first, you need to prepare one cookie sheet by using parchment paper. You may also use a baking mat (silicone).

2. Take one saucepan so that you can brown the salted butter in it on medium to high heat. Don't forget to stir often. Next, you need to stir in xanthan gum, sweetener, and heavy cream. Once you are done stirring all these ingredients, remove the pan from heat and keep it aside.

3. Meanwhile, stir in all the chopped pecans and then keep the container in the fridge for almost an hour for firming up. You will get to see that the mixture has thickened. Next, scoop out a total number of ten cookie shapes and place them on the baking sheet that you have already prepared. If you want, you may sprinkle salt. Allow the butter pralines to refrigerate until hardened.

4. Choose any air-tight container for storing and keep the container inside the refrigerator until serving.

5 pm – Sheet Pan Steak

Total Time: 50 minutes

Yields: 4

Nutrition Facts: Calories: 464 | Carbs: 26g | Protein: 42g | Fat: 22g | Fiber: 8g

Ingredients:

- One a quarter lb. of bunch broccolini (trimmed into lengths of 2 inches)
- Four finely chopped garlic cloves
- One lb. of small-sized cremini mushrooms (halved and trimmed)
- Three tbsps. of olive oil
- One 15 ounce can of cannellini beans (low-sodium and rinsed)
- A quarter tsp. of red pepper flakes
- One and a half lb. of steaks of New York strip (excess fat trimmed off)
- Pepper and Kosher salt

Method:

1. At first, the oven needs to be preheated, and for that, you need to set the temperature to exactly 450 degrees. Take one large-sized baking sheet (rimmed) and toss in broccolini, mushrooms, red pepper flakes, oil, garlic, and a quarter tsp. each of pepper and salt. After that, place your baking sheet inside the oven. All the ingredients need to be roasted for approximately fifteen minutes.

2. Next, you have to make the necessary space required for placing the steaks. For that, it is better to push the roasted mixture towards the pan's edges. Before placing the steaks in the middle of your pan, season with a quarter tsp. each of pepper and Kosher salt. Now, it is time to roast the seasoned steaks, and each side must be roasted for five to seven minutes. Roast according to your desired doneness. Then, you have to take out the roasted steaks and place them on a clean cutting board. Slice only after allowing to rest for five minutes.

3. In the meantime, keep the beans on the same baking sheet. Toss the beans for combining evenly—roast for three to four minutes until the beans are heated thoroughly. Lastly, enjoy the dish by serving vegetables and roasted beans with steak.

Day 14

11 am – High Protein Breakfast Bowl

Total time: 5 minutes

Yields: 1

Nutrition Facts: Calories: 373 | Carbs: 5g | Protein: 33g | Fat: 24g | Fiber: 5g

Ingredients:

- Three and a half ounces of cured salmon or smoked salmon
- Two large-sized boiled eggs (cut them in halves)
- Two tbsps. of cream cheese
- Three ounces of cucumber (ribboned or diced)
- A quarter lemon (cut in chunks, optional)
- Half tsp. of dried chives or bagel seasoning (optional)

Method:

1. Take a bowl of large size and place every single ingredient into it.
2. For adding extra flavor, sprinkle the required quantity of bagel seasoning. If you do not want to add bagel seasoning, then add pepper and salt.
3. Serve.

Note: In case you do not prefer salmon, you may use canned ham, deli turkey, or tuna as a substitute.

3 pm – Peanut Butter Balls

Total time: 20 minutes

Yield: 18

Nutritional Facts: Calories: 170.1 | Carbs: 7.6g | Protein: 6.4g | Fat: 14g | Fiber: 4.4mg

Ingredients:

- 1 cup of finely chopped salted peanuts, but make sure that it is not peanut flour
- 1 cup of peanut butter
- 1 cup of sweetening powder such as swerve
- 8 oz of chocolate chips (make sure that these are sugar-free)

Method:

1. Take the peanut butter, sliced peanut, and sweetener in a bowl and mix them. Now you have to divide the dough into small balls of 18 pieces. Now place these balls on a wax paper

2. Put the chocolate chips on the top of a double boiler or put it into the microwave so that it melts. But keep stirring the chocolate until they are 75% melt. Until the rest of the chocolate chips melt, keep stirring.

3. Dip those peanut butter balls into the melted chocolate and put it back on the wax paper, and refrigerate it until the chocolate becomes hard.

Note: You can use stevia leaves, xylitol, and erythritol as sweeteners, but remember that these are twice as sweet as sugar. Be careful while using these sweeteners.

5 pm – Pork Chops with Bloody Mary Tomato Salad

Total Time: 25 minutes

Yields: 4

Nutrition Facts: Calories: 400 | Carbs: 8g | Protein: 39g | Fat: 23g | Fiber: 3g

Ingredients:

- Two tsps. each of
    - Horseradish (prepared, squeezed dry)
    - Worcestershire sauce
- Two tbsps. each of
    - Red wine vinegar
    - Olive oil
- One pint of halved cherry tomatoes
- Half tsp. each of
    - Celery seeds
    - Tabasco
- Two stalks of celery (thinly sliced)
- A quarter cup of flat-leaf parsley (finely chopped)
- Four small-sized or about two and a quarter lb. of bone-in pork chops (thickness of one inch)
- Half small-sized and thinly sliced red onion
- One small head of lettuce (green-leaf, leaves torn)
- Pepper
- Kosher salt

Method:

1. Before getting ready to prepare the super delicious dish, you need to heat the grill on medium to high heat. Meanwhile, take a large-sized bowl and whisk together vinegar, oil, horseradish, celery seeds, Worcestershire sauce, Tabasco, and a quarter tsp. of salt. After the whisking is over, toss with celery, onion, and cherry tomatoes.

2. Now it is time to use half a teaspoon each of pepper and salt for seasoning pork chops and let it grill. Each side must be grilled for six to seven minutes or till the chops become golden brown and thoroughly cooked.

3. Next, you need to place the leafy parsley inside the tomatoes by folding and serve it over greens and grilled pork. You may enhance the taste by consuming it with mashed potatoes or cauliflower.

Day 15

11 am – Green Omelet

Total time: 20-25 minutes

Yields: 1

Nutrition Facts: Calories: 468 | Carbs: 4g | Protein: 21g | Fat: 41g | Fiber: 2g

Ingredients:

- Two tbsps. of fresh cilantro (finely chopped), or parsley (flat-leaf)
- Two large-sized eggs
- One green chili (finely sliced, seeded)
- Two tbsps. of whipping cream (heavy)
- Four tbsps. of cheddar cheese (shredded)
- One tbsp. of butter
- One and a quarter ounces or a cup of baby spinach or watercress (chopped roughly)
- Pepper and salt (for seasoning)

Method:

1. Take a bowl and pour the eggs into it after cracking them. Add heavy cream, green chili, and cilantro to the bowl. Use a fork for whisking all the ingredients together till the mixture combines well. Next, you need to do the seasoning with an ample quantity of pepper as well as salt as per your taste. Keep the bowl aside.

2. Now, it is time to melt one tbsp. of butter. For that, you will need a small-sized and non-stick pan. Set the flame to medium heat and place the frying pan over the burner. After melting the butter, add in the already prepared egg mixture. You have to move the eggs while it gets cooked

with the help of a spatula. Do it for nearly one minute. As soon as you notice that the exterior edges are becoming opaque, start moving the spatula all around the pan's rim. It helps in loosening the edges. In order to be sure whether the omelet is sliding or not, just shake your frying pan gently.

3. After that, all you need to do is sprinkle shredded cheese on top of the whole omelet and then the watercress. Decrease the heat and cover the pan with a lid. Leave it in this state for a few minutes. Serve after transferring the green omelet to a dish.

Note: For avoiding the spicy nature of green chili, feel free to adjust the taste by including a small lump of yogurt (thick).

3 pm – Thai Curry Soup

Total Time: 22 minutes

Yields: 6

Nutrition Facts: Calories: 323 | Carbs: 7g | Protein: 15g | Fat: 27g | Fiber: 1g

Ingredients:

Things you need for the soup

- 14.5 ounces of full-fat coconut milk
- Two teaspoons of fish sauce
- One teaspoon of honey or any other average nectar
- Four cloves of crushed garlic
- Four properly boneless and skinless chicken thighs
- Two full teaspoons of yellow Thai curry paste
- Three teaspoons of soy sauce
- One full teaspoon of honey or agave nectar

- Two finely chopped green scallion
- Two-inch of minced ginger. Chop them well.

Things you need to add to the soup after it is cooked

- Half a cup of cherry tomatoes sliced in two.
- Three finely chopped green scallions
- Juice of one lime
- One can of straw mushrooms
- One-fourth cup of chopped cilantro

Method:

For the pot,

1. Take all the ingredients for the main soup and then put them in an instant pot and seal it.
2. You need to cook the soup for about twelve minutes under pressure.
3. Release the pressure quickly and take the chicken out. Shred the chicken well and put the chicken back in the soup.
4. Now take all the veggies and add them to the broth, which is hot. Keep the veggies in the broth for some time, scalding them a little. Keep in mind to not overcook them into a mush.

For the slow cooker,

1. When you are using a slow cooker, place all the main ingredients in the cooker and cook them on low heat for about eight hours. And if you are using high heat, it should take about four hours to get cooked properly.
2. Take the veggies and put them in the cooker in the last half an hour. Keep in mind to not overcook the veggies in a mush. Just give them a little scalding so that their freshness is maintained.

3. Take out the chicken from the soup and shred it well. Then put them back in the soup.

For the stove,

1. Take a pot that has a very thick bottom and then place all the soup ingredients and the chicken in it. Cook them well till the chicken has been cooked well and the broth has become flavorful.

2. Take the chicken out and shred it properly. After you have shredded it well, place it back in the soup.

3. Take the veggies and add them to the broth that is cooking. Do not cook the veggies in mush. Give them a little scalding so that you can taste the freshness of the vegetables and the herbs.

Note: You can always substitute the heavy whipping cream with coconut milk if you want. Thai curry is also available in all the Asian stores near you. You can buy that and then cook it at home.

5 pm – Herb and Mushroom Braised Beef

Total time: 8 hours 35 minutes

Yield: 8

Nutrition Facts: Calories: 363 | Protein: 40g | Carbs: 13g | Fiber: 2g

Ingredients:

- Three pounds of chuck roast (preferably boneless). Trim and slice it into 2-inch cubes

- Two teaspoons of thinly chopped garlic

- ¼ cup of all-purpose flour

- Two teaspoons of freshly chopped thyme (keep some aside for garnishing)

- One teaspoon freshly chopped rosemary (keep some aside for garnishing)

- One teaspoon of oregano (this also should be freshly chopped)
- ¼ cup of olive oil
- 1 ½ teaspoon of kosher salt
- 8 ounces of fresh cremini mushrooms (quartered)
- 2 cups of pearl onions (preferably frozen)
- 1 ½ cups of beef stock (unsalted)
- Five medium-sized carrots, cut into 2-inch pieces (cut them diagonally)
- One tablespoon of oregano leaves (make sure that the leaves are fresh)
- One tablespoon of sherry vinegar

Method:

1. Keep the beef cubes, garlic, rosemary, thyme, flour, oregano, and ½ tablespoon of salt in a plastic zip-lock bag, seal it and then toss it to coat the beef. Take out the beef and reserve the flour mixture.

2. Heat 2 tablespoons of oil in a large pan and cook the beef until it turns brown (it will take 10 to 12 minutes).

3. Transfer this beef into a 5 to 6-quart slow cooker and reserve the dripping in the skillet.

4. Add the mushroom to the pan and cook it with the leftover oil, do not add extra oil. Keep stirring until the mushrooms turn brown (it will take around 6 to 8 minutes).

5. Now add wine to it and keep stirring. Transfer the mushrooms to the slow cooker.

6. Add beef stock, pearl onion, carrots, reserved flour mixture, one tablespoon of salt into the slow cooker, and keep stirring until everything gets mixed properly.

7. Cover and cook for 8 hours until the beef is soft and tender.

8. Now skim the fat from the cooking liquid and add vinegar to it. Keep stirring it.

9. Now that your beef is ready garnish it with the remaining chopped thyme, oregano, and rosemary.

Note: It will be better if you lock the lid and turn the pressure valve to venting. Do not rush the cooking process. You have to cook the beef slowly so that the beef becomes very tender.

Day 16

11 am – Strawberry Smoothie

Total time: 5 minutes

Yield: 2

Nutritional Facts: Calories: 416 | Carbs: 12g | Protein: 4g | Fat: 42g | Fiber: 3g

Ingredients:

- 1 ¾ cup of coconut milk (unsweetened)
- 5 oz. of strawberries (these should be fresh and slice them)
- One tablespoon of lime juice
- ½ tablespoon of vanilla extract

Method:

1. Put all the ingredients in a blender and blend until it becomes smooth.

2. If you are using canned coconut milk, then drain off the liquid and add only the creamier part to the smoothie so that your smoothie becomes creamier.

3. Add more lime juice if you want to.

Note: You can also replace coconut milk with Greek yogurt and also add two tablespoons of whey protein if you want to increase the protein value in your meal.

3 pm – Tortilla Chips

Total Time: 35 minutes

Yields: 4-6

Nutrition facts: Calories: 140 | Carbs: 21g | Protein: 1g | Fat: 7g | Fiber: 3g

Ingredients:

- One cup of almond flour
- Two cups of shredded mozzarella
- Half tsp. of chili powder
- One tsp. each of
    - Garlic powder
    - Kosher salt
- Black pepper (freshly ground)

Method:

1. First of all, preheating your oven is necessary and for that, set the temperature of your oven to exactly 35o degrees. Take two large-sized baking sheets and line them by using parchment paper.

2. After that, take one bowl (microwave safe) and use it for melting mozzarella. This might need almost a minute and thirty seconds. Then, add garlic powder, almond flour, chili powder, salt, and black pepper. You have to use your hands at this stage for kneading dough. Make sure that a soft ball is formed.

3. Once you are done kneading the dough, place it in between both the parchment paper sheets. Then, give it a rectangle shape with a thickness of one-eighth inch. Take one pizza cutter or sharp knife for cutting the dough into small triangles.

4. Next, you have to spread out the chips on the baking sheets that are already prepared and let them bake. The baking must be done for almost twelve to fifteen minutes till it begins to crisp and the edges become golden in color.

5 pm – Sweet Potato and Black Bean Burrito

Total Time: 1 hour 15 minutes

Yields: 8-12

Nutrition facts: Calories: 575.2 | Carbs: 102g | Protein: 19.8g | Fat: 10.3g | Fiber: 15.9g

Ingredients:

- Twelve flour tortillas (10 inches)
- Five cups of peeled sweet potatoes (cubed)
- Three and a half cups of diced onions
- Two tsps. of broth or two tsps. of vegetable oil
- Four pressed or minced garlic cloves
- Four tsps. each of
    - Ground coriander
    - Ground cumin
- One tbsp. of fresh and minced green chili pepper
- Two-third cup of cilantro leaf (lightly packed)
- Four and a half cups or three 15-ounce cans of black beans (drained and cooked)
- Two tbsps. of lemon juice (fresh)
- One tsp. of salt
- Fresh salsa

Method:

1. Preheat your oven and set the temperature to 350 degrees.

2. Take one medium-sized saucepan and keep the sweet potatoes in it along with water and salt to cover.

3. Cover the saucepan and let it boil. Allow the ingredients to simmer for almost ten minutes till the sweet potatoes become tender.

4. Then, you have to drain out the remaining water and keep it aside.

5. After cooking the sweet potatoes, take one medium-sized saucepan or skillet and pour oil into it. After the oil becomes warm, add in garlic, chili, and onions.

6. Cover the pan and let the ingredients cook on low-medium heat. You need to stir occasionally for almost six to seven minutes till the onions become tender.

7. Next, you need to add ground coriander and cumin to the pan. Cook for another two to three minutes, and you must not forget to stir frequently.

8. After that, set your pan aside by removing it from heat.

9. Now, it is time to take out your food processor. You have to combine cilantro, the entire quantity of black beans, salt, already cooked and tender sweet potatoes, and lemon juice in your food processor. Puree all the ingredients till it becomes perfectly smooth. In case you do not have a food processor, you may mash all the ingredients with the help of your hand by placing them in a large-sized bowl.

10. After that, take one large-sized mixing bowl for transferring the mixture of sweet potato. Mix spices and cooked onions in that mixture.

11. When you are done mixing all the ingredients, take one large-sized baking dish and oil it lightly.

12. Place two-third to a three-fourth cup of this filling inside each tortilla. Then, you need to roll the tortillas and place them in the oiled baking dish with the seam side downwards.

13. Cover the dish very tightly with the help of a foil. Let it bake for half an hour.

14. Top it with fresh salsa. Your dish is ready to be served.

Day 17

11 am – Taco Breakfast Skillet

Total Time: 1 hour

Yields: 6

Nutrition facts: Calories: 563 | Carbs: 9g | Protein: 32g | Fat: 44g | Fiber: 4g

Ingredients:

- Ten large-sized eggs
- One pound of ground beef
- Two-thirds cup of water
- Four tbsps. of Taco seasoning
- A quarter cup each of
    - Heavy cream
    - Salsa
    - Sour cream
    - Black olives (sliced)
- One and a half cups of cheddar cheese (shredded, divided)
- One medium-sized peeled avocado (cubed and pitted)
- One diced Roma tomato

- Two sliced green onions

- One sliced jalapeno (optional)

- Two tbsps. of fresh cilantro (torn, optional)

Method:

1. In the beginning, take one skillet of large size and place ground beef in it. Let the beef turn brown over medium to high heat. Drain away the extra fat.

2. Stir in water and taco seasoning to the hot skillet. Lower the heat and allow it to simmer for almost five minutes till the sauce thickens and layers the meat completely. Then, keep aside about half a portion of the beef by taking it out from the large skillet.

3. Now, take one large-sized mixing bowl for whisking the eggs after cracking them. Add a cup of cheese, heavy cream, and whisk for combining perfectly.

4. For preheating the oven, set the temperature to approximately 375 degrees.

5. In the meantime, pour the already prepared egg mixture on top of the remaining meat present in the skillet. Stir with a spatula for combining the eggs and meat. Next, you need to bake for half an hour or till it has become fluffy.

6. After the baking part is over, top it with a half cup of cheese, half portion of seasoned beef, avocado, green onion, olives, tomato, salsa, and sour cream.

7. Before serving, garnish the dish with cilantro and jalapeno.

3 pm – Keto Fat Bombs

Total time: 5 minutes

Yield: 1

Nutritional value: Calories: 194 | Fat: 16.8g | Carbs: 2g | Fiber: 1.5g | Protein: 3.8g

Ingredients:

- ½ cup of nut butter or coconut butter of your choice
- ¼ cup of melted coconut oil
- ¼ cup of cocoa or cacao powder
- One tablespoon of liquid sweetener, or you can also use stevia
- 1/8 tablespoon of salt (optional)

Method:

1. Stir all the ingredients until all ingredients become smooth (you can add coconut oil if you feel that it is very dry).
2. Now transfer it into a small container, or silicone cupcake mold, or ice cube trays, candy molds, etc., depending on your choice. Put it in the freezer till it sets.

Note: If you are using coconut oil, then make sure that you store these keto bombs in the freezer to store them.

5 pm – Pork Tenderloin with Brussels Sprouts and Butternut Squash

Total Time: 50 minutes

Yields: 4

Nutrition Facts: Calories: 401 | Carbs: 25g | Protein: 44g | Fat: 15g | Fiber: 6g

Ingredients:

- One and three-fourth lb. of trimmed pork tenderloin
- Three tbsps. of canola oil
- Two peeled cloves of garlic
- Two sprigs of fresh thyme
- Four cups each of
  - Butternut squash (diced)
  - Brussels sprouts (halved and trimmed)
- Pepper
- Salt

Method:

1. In the beginning, all you need to do is preheat your oven by setting the temperature to exactly 400 degrees. While the oven gets preheated, season the pork tenderloin properly with the required amount of pepper and salt. Take one large-sized pan of cast-iron and pour one tbsp. of oil into it. Heat the oil on medium or high heat. As you get to see that the oil is shimmering, add the seasoned tenderloin and cook for eight to twelve minutes. Sear until the tenderloin turns golden brown on all sides. Then, you need to transfer it to a large-sized plate.

2. Next, you need to add the remaining quantity of canola oil, garlic, and thyme to your pan. Cook the ingredients for almost a minute till you get their aroma. Now, it is

time to add butternut squash, brussels sprouts, and one pinch each of pepper and salt. Cook for five to six minutes by occasional stirring till all the veggies attain a slight brown color.

3. Then, you need to keep the cooked tenderloin on top of the vegetables. Transfer all the ingredients to your oven. The roasting must be done till the vegetables become tender or till your meat thermometer registers a temperature of 140 degrees when it is introduced in the tenderloin's thickest part. Roasting might take nearly fifteen to twenty minutes.

4. After that, wear oven gloves for safety and take out the hot pan from your oven very carefully. Before slicing the tenderloin, let it rest for five minutes and then serve with vegetables. You may also toss the veggies with balsamic vinaigrette before serving. Enjoy!

Day 18

11 am – Peanut Butter Chocolate Smoothie

Total time: 5 minutes

Yield: 3

Nutritional Facts: Calories: 435 | Protein: 9g | Carbs: 10g | Fat: 41g | Fiber: 4g

Ingredients:

- ¼ cup of creamy peanut butter
- 1 cup of heavy cream (you could also choose coconut milk if you want a dairy-free vegan option)
- Three tablespoons of cocoa powder
- 1 ½ cup of almond milk (do not choose a sweetened almond juice)
- Six tablespoons of best-powdered erythritol
- 1/8 tablespoon of sea salt

Method:

1. Put all the ingredients in a blender.
2. Blend until it becomes smooth.

Note: You can add a sweetener like stevia leaves, but do not use white sugar.

3 pm – Jalapeno Egg Cups

Total Time: 45 minutes

Yields: 12

Nutrition Facts: Calories: 190.58 | Carbs: 1.56g | Protein: 12.85g | Fat: 14.4g | Fiber: 0.16g

Ingredients:

- Ten large-sized eggs
- Half cup each of
  - Shredded mozzarella
  - Shredded cheddar
- A quarter cup of sour cream
- Twelve slices of bacon
- One tsp. of garlic powder
- Two jalapenos (one thinly sliced and the other one minced)
- Black pepper (Freshly ground)
- Kosher salt
- Cooking spray (non-stick)

Method:

1. For preheating your oven, set the temperature to exactly 375 degrees. Take one large-sized skillet and cook bacon in it on medium heat. The cooking must be done till the bacon attains a slight brown color and is a bit pliable. Line a plate with a paper towel and keep the cooked bacon on it to drain.

2. In the meantime, take one large-sized bowl and whisk together sour cream, eggs, minced jalapeno, garlic powder, and mozzarella, and cheddar cheese. Season all the ingredients with pepper and salt.

3. Next, you have to grease one muffin tin by using a cooking spray. Once you have finished greasing, line each cup with a bacon slice and then pour in the egg mixture. Top every single cup with one slice of jalapeno.

4. Bake for approximately twenty minutes, and the eggs must not look wet. If it looks wet, then bake for another one or two minutes. Let the egg cups cool slightly, and then remove them from the tin.

5 pm – Seared Salmon

Total Time: 40 minutes

Yields: 2

Nutrition Facts: Calories: 976 | Protein: 56g | Carbs: 7g | Fat: 80g | Fiber: 3g

Ingredients:

For the lemon sauce and salmon

- Two-thirds cup of heavy whipping cream
- Two tablespoons of fresh parsley (chop them finely)
- Juice of half a lemon
- Half teaspoon of salt
- Two tablespoons of olive oil are needed for searing
- Salt and pepper as per your taste
- Half a cup of a vegetable stalk
- One tablespoon of chives, finely chopped
- One pinch of black pepper
- Boneless fillets of salmon about 1\2" (1.2 centimeters) thick.

For serving

- Fifteen cups of fresh spinach

- Salt and pepper as per taste
- One tablespoon of butter

Method:

For the lemon sauce,

1. Take a small saucepan and then pour all the vegetables in it.
2. Over a high flame, let the vegetables boil for some time.
3. Then let it boil for some time till the stalk is reduced.
4. Then add the lemon, chives, parsley, salt, and pepper to the stalk. Whisk it for some time.
5. Reduce the heat and keep it at a low temperature. Do not cover the pan and keep whisking occasionally.
6. Let this salt get more thickened as you prepare the salmon.

For the salmon,

1. Take a large skillet or a non-stick pan.
2. Over medium to high flame heat some olive oil in it.
3. Take the pepper and the salt and season the fish on both the sides, then place it on the pan, making sure the skin side is facing down.
4. Let it sear for about four minutes till the fish is brown and crispy.
5. You need to flip the fish now; keep in mind to reduce the flame before that so that the fish does not get burnt. Cook for another three to five minutes until the fish turns golden and crispy on the outside and a light shade of pink on the inside.
6. Take a serving plate and place the fish on it. Serve hot!

For serving,

1. Take a large frying pan and add the butter. Let it melt completely over medium heat.

2. You need to add the spinach now while keeping the flame medium-high.

3. Take tongs and toss the spinach for some time in the butter. Toss it till the spinach gets wilted.

4. Add the pepper and the salt according to your taste, and remove the spinach from the pan.

5. When you are serving, make sure to squeeze some lemon juice over the salmon and serve with the sauteed spinach on the side.

Note: *Before using the salmon, let it rest for about fifteen minutes and make sure it is at room temperature. This helps the salmon to get cooked evenly. You can store the cooked salmon in your fridge for about three days. You can store the sauce in an air-tight container in your fridge for about three days. You will need to heat up the sauce well before using it every time.*

Day 19

11 am – Banana Strawberry Overnight Oats

Total time: 5 minutes

Yields: 2

Nutrition Facts: Calories: 326 | Carbs: 63g | Protein: 8g | Fat: 1g | Fiber: 7g

Ingredients:

- One and a half cups of milk (as per your choice)
- One cup of oats (old fashioned)
- A quarter cup of yogurt (strawberry flavored or plain)
- Two tbsps. of honey
- One chopped banana
- Half cup of chopped strawberries

Method:

1. First of all, take a bowl and put the oats in it. Keep it aside.
2. Now, take another bowl of medium size for whisking yogurt, milk, and honey together.
3. Once you are done whisking, pour the wet ingredients into the bowl of oats. Stirring is required for appropriately combining everything.
4. Lastly, the bananas and strawberries must be added and stirred.
5. The bowl is to be kept inside your refrigerator overnight. You may also try out an alternate option by distributing the combined mixture into one mason jar or cup before placing it inside the refrigerator. Enjoy!

Note: In case you want to have a sweeter banana strawberry overnight oat, use either vanilla or strawberry yogurt. For those who do not want it to be sweet, simply use plain yogurt.

3 pm – Burger Fat Bombs

Total Time: 30 minutes

Yields: 20

Nutrition facts: Calories: 80 | Carbs: 0g | Protein: 5g | Fat: 7g | Fiber: 0g

Ingredients:

- One lb. of ground beef
- Two tbsps. of cold butter (trimmed into twenty pieces)
- Half tsp. of garlic powder
- Two ounces of cheddar (trimmed into twenty pieces)
- Tomatoes (thinly sliced, for serving)
- Lettuce leaves (fresh, for serving)
- Mustard (needed for serving)
- Cooking spray
- Black pepper (freshly ground)
- Kosher salt

Method:

1. At first, your oven needs to be preheated at a temperature of 375 degrees. Use the required quantity of cooking spray for greasing a very small muffin tin. Then, take one medium-sized bowl and, in it, season ground beef with salt, pepper, and garlic powder.

2. Next, you need to place one tsp. of beef into each cup of the muffin tin and press it in such a manner so that it

covers the bottom completely. Keep one piece of cold butter on it, and again press one tsp. of beef so that the butter gets covered completely.

3. After that, you have to transfer one piece of cheddar into each muffin cup. Press the remaining amount of beef softly over the cheese.

4. Now, it is time for baking. Bake for about fifteen minutes and check that the meat is thoroughly cooked. Allow it to cool slightly.

5. Lastly, take one spatula (metal offset) and use it for releasing every single burger from your muffin tin. It is better to serve with mustard, tomatoes, and lettuce leaves.

5 pm – Vietnamese Pho Soup

Total time: 1 hour 15 minutes

Yield: 8

Nutritional Facts: Calories: 136 | Carbs: 4g | Protein: 14g| Fat: 6g | Fiber: 2g

Ingredients:

- One tablespoon of coconut oil
- 2-inch piece of ginger (it should be fresh, slice them)
- One onion (peel and chop it)
- Five cloves of smashed garlic
- Three whole star anise
- Four smashed cardamom pods
- Ten cloves
- 12 cups of water
- Two tablespoons of gluten-free fish sauce

- 2 cups of beef broth
- 1 pound of flank steak
- One tablespoon palm sugar
- 1 pound of shirataki noodles
- Two jalapenos (slice them)
- 4 ounces of mung bean sprouts
- One lime (cut them into wedges)
- 1 cup of basil leaves (get fresh leaves)

Method:

1. Put a large stockpot over medium heat and add ginger, onion wedges, garlic, star anise, cinnamon, cloves, cardamom, and coconut oil. Saute the onion and the spices till the onions become brown (for about 10 minutes).

2. Now pour the beef stock, sugar, fish sauce, and water into the pot and bring it to a simmer. Lower the heat and simmer it for a minimum of an hour. Also, do not skip the fish sauce. It might have a funky aroma but the taste it adds to the soup is amazing.

3. During this time, flash-freeze the flank steak for about 30 minutes. The inside should be thawed and frozen on the outside. Slice the steak into very thin pieces against the grain.

4. Pull all the onions and spices out of the broth with the help of a skimmer. On the serving plate, arrange sliced jalapeno, mung bean sprouts, lime wedges, and basil.

5. Into the broth, add noodles, and cook for 2 to 3 minutes (follow the instructions given on the package, do not overcook it).

6. Now add the thin pieces of beef to the broth after turning off the heat. The pieces of beef should be thin enough to get cooked in the hot broth without giving any additional heat.

7. Serve the pho soup into the bowls and add the veggies of your choice to garnish the soup.

Notes: You could use raw zucchini noodles or rice noodles instead of shirataki noodles. Also, cook the broth for 2 hours or more as the longer you cook the broth, the better it is for you. You could also make the broth one day before so that the flavor gets intensified before adding beef and noodles.

Day 20

11 am – Pancakes

Total time: 25 minutes

Yield: 12

Nutritional Facts: Calories: 110 | Carbs: 7g | Fiber: 3g | Fat: 6g | Protein: 11g

Ingredients:

- 1 ½ cups of wheat flour
- Two teaspoons of baking powder
- ½ teaspoon salt
- Two eggs
- Two tablespoons of any sweetener (according to your taste)
- 1 ¼ cups of milk
- Three tablespoons of vegetable oil

Method:

1. Take a large bowl and mix all the flour, baking powder, salt, and any sugar alternatives.

2. In a separate large bowl, mix eggs, oil, and milk together.

3. Now put the wet ingredients into the dry ingredients and stir and combine them. Make sure that there are no lumps, so keep stirring and mixing them until the mixture is smooth.

4. Allow the batter to rest for 10 minutes. Do not cover it.

5. Now heat a large pan over medium heat, or you can also preheat the oven at 350 degrees Fahrenheit. Lightly grease the pan with butter or vegetable oil.

6. Scoop ¼ of a cup from the batter and spread with a spoon on the pan.

7. Cook one side of the pancake properly before flipping over and cooking the other side. Make sure that the bottoms are brown and cook each side for at least 1 to 3 minutes. You could also cook for a longer time; just make sure that each side is cooked nicely.

8. Top these pancakes with any syrup of your choice.

9. If you have any leftover pancakes, wrap them properly and store them in the refrigerator.

Note: Do not use white sugar in your pancakes. Choose any other healthier sweetening options that are available in the market.

3 pm – Chocolate Mousse

Total Time: 10 minutes

Yields: 4

Nutrition facts: Calories: 218 | Carbs: 5g | Protein: 2g | Fat: 23g | Fiber: 2g

Ingredients:

- A quarter cup each of
    - Powdered sweetener
    - Cocoa powder (unsweetened, sifted)

- One cup of whipping cream (heavy)
- One tsp. of vanilla extract
- A quarter tsp. of kosher salt

Method:

1. The very first step of making chocolate mousse is whisking the entire quantity of cream till it becomes thick. For whisking, you may opt for either any hand mixer or stand mixer.

2. Next, you have to add sweetener, cocoa powder, salt, and vanilla extract. Keep whisking till the ingredients are combined smoothly.

Note: Those who are willing to make a bit lighter mousse must whisk the egg whites of three large-sized eggs to firm peaks. Then, it must be folded into your mousse mixture for combining as required.

5 pm – Fresh Spinach Frittata

Total Time: 45 minutes

Yields: 4

Nutrition Facts: Calories: 695 | Carbs: 5g | Protein: 34g | Fat: 60g | Fiber: 2g

Ingredients:

- Two tablespoons of butter
- Eight eggs
- One and forth cups of cheddar cheese, shredded
- Salt and pepper
- Chorizo or diced bacon (five-ounce of diced bacon)
- Seven and a half cups of fresh spinach (eight-ounce of fresh spinach)

- One full cup of a heavy whipping cream

Method:

1. At first, you need to set the temperature of the oven to 350 degrees Fahrenheit and preheat.

2. Next, you need to grease a baking dish of about nine by nine or use individual ramekins.

3. In the next step, you need to fry the bacon in the butter, keeping the heat medium. Fry until it is crispy. When the bacon has become crispy, go on to add the fresh spinach and stir it well until it has wilted.

4. Now take the pan off the heat and let it cool down.

5. Take the eggs and whisk them really well with the fresh cream. When you are done whisking them well, pour them into the dish you are using for baking or in the ramekins.

6. After this, keep adding the spinach, cheese, and bacon on top of it. Bake this for twenty-five minutes to half an hour. Bake it till it is completely st in the middle and has gotten a nice golden color on top.

Notes: What will absolutely make this dish go on another level is if you serve some shredded cabbage and greens on the side along with some homemade dressing. Enjoy!

Day 21

11 am – Bacon and Avocado Eggs

Total time: 60-65 minutes

Yields: 2

Nutrition Facts: Calories: 407 | Carbs: 2g | Protein: 25g | Fat: 31g | Fiber: 2.3g

Ingredients:

- Four large-sized eggs
- One tsp. of olive oil
- Two and a half ounces of bacon
- Three and a half ounces of avocado
- Pepper and salt

Method:

1. At first, the oven needs to be preheated by setting the temperature to 350 degrees. You may use aluminum foil or parchment paper for lining one baking sheet (rimmed). After lining the sheet, spread the strips of bacon on it. Keep it aside.

2. Take one saucepan and place all the eggs in it and then fill it up with almost cold water. The level of water must be at least an inch above the eggs. Cover the saucepan with a lid and let it boil lightly by setting the flame to high heat. Remove the saucepan from your burner as soon as it begins to boil properly. Keep the pan covered for about fifteen minutes so that the eggs rest inside it. After that, pour ice-cold water into a bowl and place all the eggs in it with the help of one slotted spoon. Let the eggs stay in this manner for five to ten minutes. You may also try another option- keep the boiled eggs in one

colander and place it under running cold water till the eggs cool completely. Peel them and keep them aside.

3. Now, it is time to set the already lined baking sheet on your oven's middle rack for cooking the bacon for almost ten to twenty minutes. It is better to cook till the bacon becomes crispy, and the time may vary as it entirely depends upon the bacon's thickness. Once done, use paper towels for draining slices of bacon. For forming the sails, the cooled bacon needs to be cut into medium-sized triangles.

4. Then, slice the boiled eggs lengthwise. Use a spoon to take out the egg yolks. Place the scooped yolks, olive oil, and avocado in one small-sized bowl. Use a fork for mashing the ingredients of the bowl until combined. For enhancing the taste, you may season with pepper and salt.

5. Lastly comes the assembling part. Spoon the yolk and avocado mixture into the sliced egg whites very generously. Place the sails of bacon in the mixture's center. Serve and enjoy!

3 pm – Corn Fritters

Total time*:* 20 minutes

Yield: 4

Nutritional Facts: Calories: 274 | Fat: 28g | Protein: 3g | Carbs: 1g | Fiber: 0g

Ingredients:

- 3 ½ oz. of cauliflowers (cut them into florets)
- Two tablespoons of coconut flour
- One teaspoon of anise or fennel seeds
- ½ cup of coconut oil
- One egg

- ¼ teaspoon of salt

Method:

1. Pulse the cauliflower in a food processor until the texture becomes like coarse cornmeal or has a texture of polenta.

2. Take a big bowl and mix the eggs, cauliflower, coconut flour, anise seeds, and salt with a spatula until everything gets mixed properly.

3. Heat some oil in a small frying pan over medium heat.

4. Scoop out tablespoons of cauliflower into the frying oil but make sure not to put more than three scoops at once.

5. Fry them until they turn golden brown on both sides. Make sure that you are cooking both sides evenly.

6. Place these on a paper towel to remove extra oil after frying them properly. Serve hot.

Note: Make sure that you remove the excess oil and use the paper towels.

5 pm – Chicken with Cauliflower Rice

Total time: 35 minutes

Yield: 4

Nutritional Facts: Calories: 305 | Carbs: 12.2g | Fat: 15.5g | Protein: 29.9g | Fiber: 3g

Ingredients:

- Two large eggs (eggs should be beaten)
- Three thinly sliced scallions (separate the greens and whites)
- One teaspoon of peanut oil and two tablespoons of the same oil and keep them separately
- One tablespoon of chopped garlic
- One tablespoon of freshly grated ginger

- 1 pound of boneless, skinless chicken thigs, trim them, and cut them into 1/2-inch pieces
- 1 cup of trimmed and halved snow peas
- ½ cup of red bell pepper (dice them)
- 4 cups of cauliflower rice
- One teaspoon of sesame oil
- Three tablespoons of soy sauce or reduced-sodium tamari

Method:

1. Take a large flat-bottomed cooking ware or a large, heavy skillet, put one teaspoon of oil in it, and heat it over high heat. Add eggs to the heated oil and do not stir until one side is cooked fully; it will take about 30 minutes. Flip and cook the other side too and transfer to a cutting board and cut into ½ inch pieces.

2. Now add one tablespoon of oil into the pan and add garlic, ginger, scallion whites. Once that is done, keep stirring them until they are cooked and the scallions are soft, cook for about 30 seconds.

3. Cook for a minute after you added the chicken as well. Add snow peas and bell pepper and keep stirring until everything becomes tender (cook for at least 2 to 4 minutes). Remove everything from the pan and transfer it to another large bowl

4. Now that your pan is empty again, add one tablespoon of oil into the pan, add cauliflower and keep stirring until the cauliflowers soften (cook for about 2 minutes)

5. Now add the eggs and chicken mixture to the pan, and add tamari or soy sauce and also a bit of sesame oil and keep stirring until everything gets mixed well. Garnish with scallion leaves and serve hot

Note: You could look for cauliflower rice in the market as well. Or you could also look for other vegetable rice options in the supermarket.

Made in the USA
Coppell, TX
30 January 2022